WILLIAM HARVEY

William Harvey

A Life in Circulation

Thomas Wright

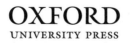

OXFORD
UNIVERSITY PRESS

Oxford University Press is a department of the
University of Oxford. It furthers the University's
objective of excellence in research, scholarship,
and education by publishing worldwide.

Oxford   New York
Auckland Cape Town Dar es Salaam Hong Kong Karachi
Kuala Lumpur Madrid Melbourne Mexico City Nairobi
New Delhi Shanghai Taipei Toronto

With offices in
Argentina Austria Brazil Chile Czech Republic France Greece
Guatemala Hungary Italy Japan Poland Portugal Singapore
South Korea Switzerland Thailand Turkey Ukraine Vietnam

First published in the United States of America in 2013 by Oxford University Press
198 Madison Avenue, New York, New York 10016

www.oup.com

Oxford is a registered trade mark of Oxford University Press in the UK and certain other countries.

Library of Congress Cataloging-in-Publication Data
Wright, Thomas (Thomas Edward), 1973–
William Harvey: a life in circulation/Thomas Wright.
p.   cm.
"Originally published, in a slightly different format, as Circulation :
William Harvey's revolutionary idea, in Great Britain
by Chatto & Windus, 2012"—T.p. verso.
Includes bibliographical references and index.
ISBN 978-0-19-993169-9
(acid-free paper) 1. Harvey, William, 1578–1657.
2. Physicians—England—Biography. 3. Physiologists—England—Biography.
4. Anatomists–England–Biography.
5. Human anatomy—England—History—17th century. 6. Blood—Circulation—History—17th
century. 7. Medicine—England—History—17th century. 8. Science—England—History—17th century.
9. England—Intellectual life—17th century. I. Wright, Thomas (Thomas Edward), 1973– Circulation.
II. Title.
QP26.H3W75   2013
610.92—dc23
[B]
2012008754

1 3 5 7 9 8 6 4 2
Printed in the United States of America
on acid-free paper

For S. G., *cor cordium*

Contents

Use of the poetic faculty in science?

Rem[ember] how the early Greeks had mystic anticipations of nearly all great modern scientific truths: the problem really is what place has imagination and the emotions in science: and primarily rem[ember] that man must use all his faculties in the search for truth: in this age we are so inductive that our facts are outstripping our knowledge—there is so much observation, experiment, analysis—so few wide conceptions . . . we want more ideas and [fewer] facts: the magnificent generalizations of Newton and Harvey c[oul]d never have been completed in this mod[ern] age where eyes are turned to earth and particulars.

Oscar Wilde, *Oxford Notebooks*

Preface

IN 1628 WILLIAM Harvey published his revolutionary 'circulation' theory of the movement of the blood. The theory demolished centuries of anatomical and physiological orthodoxy, and introduced a radical conception of the workings of the human body that had profound cultural consequences, influencing economists, poets and political thinkers. Its impact on what we now call the 'history of science', and on general culture, was, in its way, arguably as great as Darwin's theory of evolution and Newton's theory of gravity.

Harvey was one of the great heroes of the English Renaissance. He illuminated England with the flame of continental learning, having acquired the basis of his intellectual vision at Padua University. In the process, he became famous among his discerning contemporaries as the first Englishman to be deeply 'curious in Anatomie', and the first to make vivisections of 'Frogges, Toades, and a number of other Animals'. He was also revered as the only man in history who lived to see his revolutionary idea gain wide currency.

Yet despite all this, Harvey is not as well known as many other English 'scientists' (to use a nineteenth century term), or indeed as many other notable English men and women of his period. His life, and the story of his quest to understand the movement of the blood and the function of the heart, deserve to be better known.

William Harvey tells that story—it is the biography of an idea as much as it is the biography of a man.

Born of Kentish yeoman stock, William Harvey had two great ambitions: worldly advancement and intellectual immortality. These aims were closely linked for him, just as they were for William Shakespeare. For both these sons of the English yeomanry, intellectual achievement offered the only accessible route to social progress. Harvey's twin ambitions were related in a practical sense as well: it was only when he had achieved material success, and established his name as a physician, that he could buy time for his researches and gain an audience for his theory. His unconventional ideas would have been disregarded had they not been endorsed by the President of the College of Physicians, or by his beloved patron, King Charles I.

Harvey's rise through the professional and social ranks provides the background to my account of his private anatomical studies. His worldly progress is outlined in Part I, along with his intellectual formation. The story of his quest proper begins in Part II, where Harvey's countless 'experiments' (as we would call them) on human corpses and live animals are described, and the development of his revolutionary idea is charted.

Harvey's experiments—the cutting and the observing—were crucial to his theory. Yet I believe that Harvey's most important work was done not by his hands and eyes, but by his brain. We must always remember that Harvey was a natural philosopher, engaged in an overtly *philosophical* endeavour, rather than a prototype of the modern inductive scientist, dressed in doublet and hose rather than a lab coat. We should also bear in mind that the circulation theory was far from self-evident in his time, and that it could not be demonstrated to the senses. Men could no more see blood coursing around their arteries and veins, going to and from the heart, than they could perceive that the earth was spinning round. Neither did the theory have the weight of 'empirical' evidence on its side (and in any case, empirical evidence was not the litmus test of truth in the seventeenth century). Harvey's theory was born (and would have to triumph) as a philosophical idea.

The Harvey who paces through the pages of this book is a thinker—and, more specifically, a seventeenth-century thinker. His mind was incredibly sensitive to the intellectual and cultural spirit of his age, and his ideas were expressive of that spirit. That is why I have placed his work in the broader scholarly, cultural and social context of his time, in a series of thematic essays interspersed between the chronological chapters. In some of these I compare Harvey's ideas to those of contemporary poets, playwrights, economists, alchemists and preachers, and consider their possible influence on his theory; in others I look at how London, and seventeenth-century technology, shaped his thinking. The essays conjure up the late Renaissance world that Harvey inhabited; they also offer the reader an opportunity to wander around a remarkable seventeenth-century mind, and to enter into a dialogue with a culture that is rich and strange.

One of the unfamiliar things about seventeenth-century intellectual culture is its homogeneity: while science and the humanities today form two separate, highly specialized cultures, at that time a theologian could understand an astronomer without much difficulty, and law students and poets attended anatomical lectures. A broad sympathy—based on a shared language and a common set of ideas and aims—connected every discipline. These concepts and metaphors formed the landscape of Harvey's imagination, and determined the movements of his mind. They shaped and prompted his circulation theory, which grew organically, though not fully formed, out of the culture of the period.

Many of Harvey's research papers were destroyed by a wilful act of political vandalism during the English Civil War. Some of the manuscripts compiled after that date went up in the flames of the Great Fire of 1666, along with his personal library. Nevertheless there are plenty of alternative primary sources available, and these provide the foundation for the educated conjectures I make about his investigations. Did Harvey use his servants as guinea pigs for his experiments? There is no way of knowing, but other natural philosophers of the period did (Robert Boyle went so far as to administer poison to his), so I have suggested that Harvey followed the general rule. What did Harvey's private research chamber look like? We do not know, but from references in Harvey's writings, and the descriptions of the rooms of other natural philosophers, I have built an imaginative reconstruction.

All of the dramatized episodes that appear in this book have been fashioned from surviving sources. My account of Harvey's public dissection has, for example, been recreated from his manu-script lecture notes, his published works, eyewitness reports of contemporary dissections, various sixteenth- and seventeenth-century manuals for anatomists, and the letters he exchanged with members of his audiences and with other anatomists. In my depic-tion of this, and all the other set piece scenes in the book, I have invented nothing; every detail is derived from primary evidence.

One final point. While this book contains various accounts of experiments on living animals, it is by no means intended as a general and personal endorsement of the practice of animal vivisection.

Prologue. A new theory (1636): 'Blood moves . . . in a circle, continuously'

IN THE SPRING of 1636, William Harvey, physician to Charles I of England, was sent to the Continent by his king as part of a diplomatic mission to the Holy Roman Emperor Ferdinand II. Towards the end of May the English party arrived in Nuremberg, a city where Harvey's name was known to the medical establishment. It was arranged for him to give an anatomical lecture at the nearby University of Altdorf, so that he might demonstrate his controversial theory of the circulation of blood.

On 18 May, the diminutive English anatomist, draped in a billowing white gown and with a round white bonnet fixed on his broad head, entered the anatomical theatre at the university. As he walked over to the wooden dissection table, Harvey's steps were short, and a little tentative, on account of his being often troubled with gout. On the table various anatomical instruments had been laid out; a chair for the lecturer stood behind it.

The crowd were standing in rows, the president of the university and the higher-ranking professors at the front, members of the general public crammed in together at the back. Harvey looked out at feathered hats, beards, caps, gowns and expectant faces.

The audience in turn gazed back at a round-faced Englishman, with a wispy moustache and an angular chin, barely covered by a thin, pointed beard. Harvey's face was still smooth and youthful; his stature and energetic demeanour also made him seem much younger than his fifty-eight years. Beneath the large bonnet, his raven-black hair, now flecked with white, was visible in one or two places, with a curl dangling over his left ear. The tail end of the large vein that throbbed on Harvey's temple could also just be seen.

Harvey's skin was of an 'olivaster' or 'olive' complexion; friends compared it to 'the colour of wainscot'. His cheeks flushed deep red when he was cogitating or whenever his passions were roused—which was often, as he was a notoriously choleric 'hott-head'. Flashes of Harvey's emotions, and of his lightning-quick mind, were discernible in his 'little Eies', which were 'round, very black, full of spirit'.

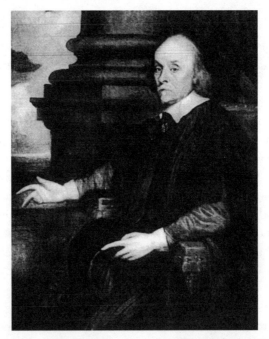

In this portrait, painted some years after the Altdorf demonstration, Harvey's beady eyes still sparkle. Large eyebrows canopy them, the left eyebrow typically raised higher than the right, giving him a permanently quizzical expression.

The Englishman was known to his audience as the author of the Latin volume *Exercitatio anatomica de motu cordis et sanguinis in animalibus*, which had been published in 1628 (the title was translated as *Anatomical Exercises Concerning the Motion of the Heart and the Blood in Living Creatures*; hereafter referred to as *De motu cordis*). This little book, in which Harvey propounded his theory of the motion of the heart and the circulation of the blood, had made him a famous, and divisive, figure across Europe. While some younger anatomists were open to his radical and innovative ideas, Harvey attracted hostile criticism from much of the medical establishment. His demonstration at Altdorf was part of a long campaign to gain acceptance for his theory, it being especially important that he convinced universities with prestigious medical and anatomical faculties.

Harvey addressed his Altdorf audience in Latin, the common linguistic currency of Europe, and the language of scholarship. 'I will demonstrate to you today', he announced, 'how blood is sent from the heart throughout the body via the aorta by means of the heartbeat. Having nourished the remotest parts of the body, the blood flows back to the veins from the arteries, then returns to its original source, the heart. The blood moves in such a quantity around the body and with so vigorous a flow that it can only move in a circle, continuously. This is an entirely new theory but, as you will learn, numerous arguments and our senses confirm that it is true.'

The men on the front rows, learned in anatomy, medicine and natural philosophy, felt the full force of the claim. Harvey's declaration represented an unprecedentedly direct and comprehensive challenge to orthodox views on the function of the heart and the motion of the blood, which had been established in Roman times. If accepted, the theory would constitute the most momentous development in anatomy (the study of the bodily structure of humans and animals) and physiology (the study of the functions of living organisms and their parts) since the second century AD. The textbooks would have to be rewritten, traditional medical therapy re-evaluated.

While Harvey had been speaking, porters of the university led a dog into the theatre. Lifting the animal up on to the dissection table, they tied its jaws shut with some rope so that it could not bite or howl. Then they pinned it down on its back and forced its limbs apart, tying its paws to four wooden stakes on the table, so that it lay spreadeagled.

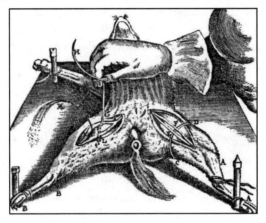

A seventeenth-century illustration of the vivisection of a dog. Vivisection, a Latinate word meaning 'the cutting of the living', was coined in the eighteenth century.

'It is obviously easier', Harvey commented, by way of explaining the dog's arrival, 'to observe the movement and function of the heart in living animals than in dead men'. Then he took a knife from the table, moved forward, and bent over the animal. With a determined thrust he plunged the blade into the dog's thorax. As he did so his sleeves became splattered with blood, while the dog writhed violently beneath him in appalling pain.

Having successfully laid bare the beating heart, Harvey put down his knife, and picked up a rod. With this he indicated the rising and falling of the dog's heart. 'You can see', he commented, 'that the heart's active phase is contraction: when it drives out the blood as it were by force, as I shall now demonstrate.' Harvey lay his rod on the table, and took up his knife once again: 'While the dog's heart is still beating', he continued, 'we will see what happens if one of the arteries is cut or punctured during the tensing of the heart.' Harvey held his knife over the dog's pulmonary artery, waiting for the moment when the heart was in contraction; then, in one sure and quick movement, he cut the artery and stepped back.

The dog's blood 'spurted forth with great force and raging ran forth in a headlong stream' (on occasion it travelled as far as three or four feet away from the animal, showering spectators in the front row). Amidst the tumult that invariably ensued, Harvey remained calm, and asked the audience to observe how the blood continued to gush out of the dog's heart when it contracted. He also asked them to note the force of the expulsion and the copious amount of liquid expelled, adding that even a conservative estimate of that quantity would have to be multiplied by seventy-two (the average heart rate), and then by sixty, to arrive at the average amount of blood discharged by the heart in an hour.

The uproar of the audience would have eventually subsided, along with the dog's dying groans and convulsions. Harvey put down his knife before delivering his conclusion. 'Calculations of the amount of blood leaving the heart and visual demonstrations of its force, confirm my supposition; I am therefore obliged to conclude that in animals the blood is driven round in a circuit with an unceasing circular movement, and that this is an activity or function of the heart which it carries out by virtue of its pulsation.' And with that, the small Englishman retired to his seat.

PART I:
RAISING HIMSELF FROM THE GROUND

1. A Kentish upbringing (1578–1593): 'Half Farmer and half Gentleman'

THOMAS HARVEY (1549–1623), William's father, came from a long line of industrious and prosperous sheep farmers, who owned property and land around Folkestone. The Harveys were proud of their birthplace and their well-to-do yeoman status. Kentish men, famed for their courage and independence, formed a cohesive and immediately identifiable regional group. So singular were they that they were popularly believed to possess tails (a legend possibly derived from their heroic defence of England during the invasion of William the Conqueror, when they reputedly dragged trees behind them, then lifted them above their heads to threaten the French). When the rich twang of the Kentish accent, and their characteristic addition of the letter 'o' to words (transforming 'my', into 'moi', 'going' into 'gooing' etc.) was heard in the taverns of the English capital, Londoners would mimic the 'long-Kentish-tailed' speaker.

Yeomen, who were officially defined as 'freemen born English' depending 'on their own free land in yearly revenue to the sum of [at least] forty shillings', constituted a no less homogeneous and recognizable class. Their defining attribute was honesty, a combination of integrity and candour, solidity and stolidity. 'Yeoman's bread', which contained only native bran, may have been rougher than foreign bread but it was more honest, being both tasty and filling. Honesty also denoted diligence: 'Being a good housekeeper', a social commentator wrote, the yeoman 'is an honest man; and so he rises early in the morning; and being up, he hath no end of motion, but wanders in his woods so continually that when he sleeps or sits, he wanders also'. As these virtues were seen as quintessentially English, yeomen came to be regarded as emblems of the nation. They were the 'filling stones' in the wall of the English Commonwealth, the very 'pith and substance of the country'.

From character sketches of William Harvey later penned by his aristocratic acquaintances, the doctor emerges as an archetypal yeoman. One noble friend christened him 'Ye little perpetual mov[ement] Dr Heruye', because of his boundless energy and unquenchable desire to 'satisfy his curiosity'—Harvey would, he said, always be 'making excursions into the Woods where he was like to be lost' in order to make 'Observations of strange Trees, and plants, and earths etc.' The same aristocrat also referred to the physician as the 'little *honest* Doctor Hervey'; nor was he the only courtier to allude to this yeoman virtue. Another praised Harvey's 'discreate and honest caryage . . . and his parents and friends are so honest people, as I dare (and that without darine) venter lyfe and lymme for him'.

Yeomen, it was said, 'have a certain pre-eminence, and more estimation than . . . the rascabilitie [i.e.] husbandmen [tenant farmers], labourers, and the lowest sort of people . . . yeomen are also for the most part farmers to gentlemen, and with grazing [and] frequenting of markets . . . do come to great wealth, insomuch that many are able and do buy the lands of unthrifty gentlemen'. Although the popular saying had it that the yeoman of Kent was 'half Farmer and half Gentleman', the odds were against him ever being absorbed fully into ranks of the aristocracy.

According to sixteenth-century preachers, 'God hath appointed every man his degree and office, within the limits whereof it behoveth him to keep himself.' Many gentlemen of the period maintained that 'Those who rushed upon professions and ways of life unequal to their natures, dishonour not only themselves . . . but pervert the harmony of the whole world.' Conservative elements of the establishment wanted to restrict social mobility, proposing a limit on the amount of land yeomen could purchase, as well as a cap on the number of yeomen's sons entering the Inns of Court, the gateway to the legal profession.

Yet despite such schemes, the sixteenth century was a propitious time for upward mobility, offering numerous opportunities to the enterprising, and where there was a will there was often a way. As a result of a sharp population increase, the more ambitious and fortunate yeomen profited, exploiting new markets, at the expense of those lower down the social scale.

Clergymen held that self-interest and social interest were incompatible, condemning as immoral self-made men who amassed personal fortunes. Thomas Harvey, however, had no qualms about getting on. Capitalizing on Folkestone's proximity to the Continent, and its extensive national and international trading links, he used the family coffers to found a courier service for goods and letters, which he circulated across Southern England and France. Profits from his business, along with the revenue he drew from the extensive Harvey lands and properties, amounted to a sum well over the annual forty shillings entitling him to yeomanly status. Thomas occupied an exalted position within the yeoman class, as did many of his fellow Kentishmen, who were popularly believed to 'bear the bell for wealth from all the yeoman rank in England'.

By 1575, the twenty-five-year-old had accumulated enough money to secure an excellent match in the marriage market, wedding Juliana Halke (or Hawke). Following her sudden death a year later, Thomas immediately formed an alliance with one of her cousins, Joan. Although they were not of aristocratic status, the Halkes were wealthy enough to warrant a brass plaque in their local church, at Hasting-Leigh, adorned with their family emblem, the hawk.

Thomas may also have worshipped at Hasting-Leigh, where Joan's father was a churchwarden. Attendance at church was compulsory on Sundays, on pain of a 12d fine, under Queen Elizabeth's 1558 Acts of Uniformity and Supremacy. These Acts had re-established the Protestant Church of England (founded by Elizabeth's father Henry VIII) with the monarch at its head, following the five-year reign of Queen Mary (1553–1558), during which the country had reverted to its 'Old Faith', Catholicism. The Harveys seem to have successfully negotiated the violent religious vicissitudes, and hostilities, of the period. Thomas certainly had no difficulty conforming to the Elizabethan dispensation, orthodoxy with regard to the next world being a requisite for those who wished to succeed in this one. Not that his attitude to religion was cynical—like all of the Harveys (William included), Thomas sincerely held the broad Christian beliefs of the time, concerning divine providence, the afterlife, and God's creation and continuing guidance of the natural world. It is likely that Thomas listened dutifully, even approvingly, to the official sermons that issued from the country pulpit, typically delivered 'against idleness', 'un-cleanliness' and 'excess of Apparel'.

On 1 April 1578, Thomas and Joan's first son William was born in Folkestone in a 'faire-built stone' house known as the post-house, which was probably the headquarters of Thomas' flourishing business operations. Mrs Harvey, a 'Godly harmless woman', and a 'charitable quiet Neighbour' (according to a brass tablet placed in the parish church on her death) matched her husband's industry, and lived up to her reputation as a 'provident diligent Huswyfe', by bearing him six further sons and two daughters.

Nothing is known about Harvey's childhood, but it is possible to imagine aspects of it from his later life. As an adult, he saw nature in microscopic detail, and was endlessly curious about its operations—and in such cases (the most famous example being Leonardo da Vinci) the child is often father of the man. He gazed intently at spiders, as they were, in the words of his writings, 'borne

through the air by an invisible thread spun from their own bodies';
he listened to the 'neighing of horses' and noted how the attendant
'motion agitated' their diaphragms; he measured the tongues of
dogs, and laughed as they 'rolled about and scratched themselves';
he was fascinated by the animation of animals in coitus, and amused
to see them quite 'crestfallen' and 'pin-buttockt'd' after the event.
He was both drawn to, and repelled by, the strong smell of animal
excrement; he felt impelled to put his hand inside the carcass of
a pig, to feel the 'buttery, oyly' texture of its fat. He was knowledgeable about hens' eggs, and, after patient study, could tell 'which
hen in a flock had lain a given egg'.

Young William must have delighted in observing such marvels
on his jaunts through the rolling hills, cherry-filled orchards and
hayfields of Kent, famed as the 'garden of England'. The boy was
doubtless drawn to the sea too, and to its myriad creatures, learning
how to identify the various molluscs which clung to the sandstone
rocks that cup Folkestone's beach, and how to 'flatter' the 'cunning'
trout there 'into destruction with an angle'.

The mature Harvey retained the country-boy's idiomatic and
colourful manner of speech, often uttering curses such as 'damme'.
His 'ordinary drink', a friend said, 'whereof he used to drink much',
was 'pleasant Water-Cider', a classic Kentish yeoman's beverage,
which Harvey himself brewed. 'Take one bushel of Pippins,' his recipe
went, 'cut them into slices . . . boil them till the goodness of them
be in the water . . . put a point of Ale-yeast to it, and set it working
two nights and days . . . till the yeast fall dead at the top . . . Within
a fortnight you may drink of it.' Here the voice of Harvey's childhood
can be heard, speaking the language and lore of Kent.

Harvey's father had two aims in life: to raise himself (and thereby
his sons) to the status of a gentleman, and to see his boys become
wealthier than himself and any of their forebears. Gentlemanly
status was often difficult to secure—an official government grant
of the right to bear a coat of arms being a prerequisite. The acquisition of arms, according to a commentator, 'set upon [the yeoman]

like an ague . . . it breaks [his] sleep, takes away his stomach, and he can never be quiet till the herald hath given him the cuckoo . . . or some ridiculous emblem for his arms. The bringing up and marriage of his eldest son is an ambition which afflicts him as soon as the boy is born, and the hope to see his son superior . . . drives him to dote upon the boy in his cradle.'

The eldest son bore the full burden of his father's expectations. While his brothers would be bound as apprentices in trade, a step that involved relatively little expense for the head of the household, William was instead bred to learning. Education was costly but Thomas was determined that his firstborn advance in the world, and he knew that his best hope of doing so lay through study. Sending their eldest sons to school was a characteristic strategy of yeomen who defied the common prejudice that knowledge of husbandry, and Scripture, was more than enough for their offspring. Gentlemen, as well as preachers, fulminated against the foundation of grammar schools, which catered for 'the vulgar sort, who be subject [only] to obey'.

Nevertheless grammar schools proliferated in the sixteenth century, nurturing the minds of countless 'upstarts' and 'mushrooms' from the yeoman class such as William Shakespeare.* The nearest grammar school to Folkestone was the King's School in Canterbury, which had been established in the middle of the century for the benefit of 'fifty poor boys, both destitute of the aid of friends and endowed with minds born and apt for learning'. 'Let the poor man's child', the statutes read, 'enter the [school] room'; William Harvey entered it in 1588, at around the age of ten.

---

* Harvey evidently recognized the importance of grammar schools, both for himself and for the commonwealth as a whole. He would later found his own grammar school, leaving money in his will for the establishment of a sizeable institution in Folkestone. The school was founded in 1674 by his nephew, Sir Eliab Harvey, executor of Harvey's estate. The Harvey Grammar School for Boys is one of only 150 or so state-funded secondary education grammar schools that remain open in England today.

At King's Harvey learned a little Greek and a smattering of Hebrew. The focus of the lessons was Latin—the language in which most of them were taught, and in which the student had to respond at all times. The school day began at six, opening with lengthy prayers, followed by long lessons until seven in the evening. During classes any inattention was punished with a severe beating. 'If any . . . boy', the statutes read, 'be remarkable for extraordinary slowness and dullness [he will be] expelled and another substituted that he may not like a drone devour the honey of the bees.' Mealtimes offered a welcome break, but little in the way of pleasure: the frugal diet consisted of milk, eggs, bread, butter and a little meat.

William is unlikely to have complained about the exacting academic demands, the regimented school life, or the food; it is impossible to picture him as Shakespeare's 'whining schoolboy', creeping 'like a snail unwillingly to school'. He had been brought up strictly, and no doubt on honest yeoman fare. In any case, to have complained would have been tantamount to disobeying his father, and a sixteenth-century son was expected to obey his father in all things. On encountering Thomas, in public as well as in private, it was customary for William to kneel down and ask his father's blessing.

With the encouragement of Thomas, and the support of a family renowned in the community for its solidarity, Harvey excelled at school. He convinced the schoolmasters (and, more importantly, his father) that he had the requisite industry and intelligence to embark on a university degree, and could justify the expense this would entail. At the age of fifteen William became the first ever Folkestone Harvey to attend university.

2. Cambridge studies I (1593): 'Making low legs to a nobleman'

WILLIAM HARVEY STOOD in front of the entrance to Gonville and Caius College in Cambridge High Street, towards the end of May 1593. It was a simple arch, adorned with Corinthian capitals, called Porta Humilitatis, the Gate of Humility. Walking beneath it, the new arrival was confronted by a far more imposing gate, the Gate of Virtue (Porta Virtutis), the entrance to the college courts and chambers. Harvey reached it via Tree Court, an avenue of young trees planted three decades previously.

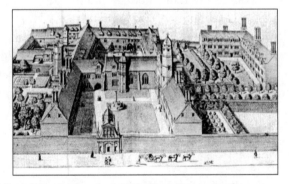

Caius College, Cambridge (c. 1690). Tree Court can be seen on the right; the Gate of Virtue stands under the tall, central tower and offers access to the spacious quadrangle, Caius Court.

The Gate of Virtue's facade, on its eastern side, is embellished with a series of Ionic, Corinthian and composite pilasters.

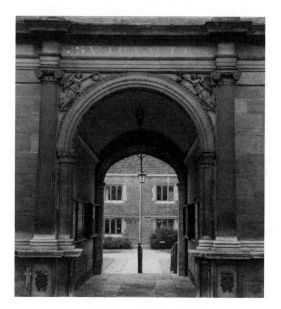

The Gate of Virtue, with its two sculptures of the Goddess Fortune: to the left of the arch she holds a palm and a laurel wreath, denoting glory, to the right a cornucopia and a bag of gold, symbolizing worldly success.

Passing under the gate, and so through into Caius Court, Harvey could look back at the gate's less elaborate western face, which is adorned with a Latin inscription to wisdom.

In the centre of Caius Court there was a stone column, which supported a weathercock in the shape of Pegasus, the winged horse that leaped out of the spurting blood of the decapitated Medusa. The column boasted sixty sundials. There were six more sundials on the hexagonal turret of the most ornate of all the college gates—the Gate of Honour (Porta Honoris), located on the south side of the court (visible in the foreground of the engraving on the previous page). Designed in the style of a High Renaissance triumphal arch, the gate has pilasters and a pediment; it is embellished with intricate circular symbols.

The Gate of Honour marked the last stage of the intellectual journey that each Caius student was encouraged to complete. Having adopted a humble attitude to their studies on arrival at the college, and having lived virtuous and wise lives during their time there, they would be ready to receive the honour of a degree. That degree would be conferred upon them during an elaborate ceremony in the Old (examination) Schools, which lay just beyond the Gate of Honour. No student was permitted to pass under the gate before the day of his graduation.*

The layout of the college is a symbolic fantasy designed by its second founder, the physician, anatomist and humanist John Caius (1510– 1573). Originally established in 1348 as Gonville Hall by the rector Edmund Gonville, Cambridge's fourth oldest college was re-founded by Caius, under the name of Gonville and Caius, in 1557. On becoming master of the comparatively small Cambridge institution in 1559, Caius set about raising its status, bestowing on it twenty scholarships during his reign. Along with the famous gates, Caius also built the Court, which was named after him, and in which Harvey stood on his first day.

Apart from the Gate of Honour, the south side of Caius Court had been left entirely free from architectural features. The chapel is on the north side, rooms on the east and west, but in the south it was decreed by the college that no building block out the sun, or prevent the 'circulation of air, which might damage the health of those dwelling [there] and speed the coming of illness and death'. The circulating air and the sunshine were especially refreshing in May, the month being renowned for the sweetness of its air, which was believed to make men merry.

---

* Many modern-day Caius students still refuse to pass through the Gate of Honour until they have completed their degrees. In the twentieth century students contributed to the venerable tradition of giving the college gates abstract names, by adding a 'fourth gate' to the scheme, between Tree Court and Gonville Court. Allowing immediate access to the lavatories, it was christened the 'Gate of Necessity'.

On that May day in 1593, whatever merriness Harvey may have felt would have been mingled with exhaustion and hunger. After an arduous journey up from Kent, he must have been as famished as the playwright Christopher Marlowe (another Kentish-born Cantabrian, and former King's School, Canterbury student) who had completed the same trip thirteen years previously. On arrival at his college Marlowe wolfed down a penny meal in hall consisting of beef, oatmeal porridge and a few 'cues' (tiny portions) of beer.

In the days following his arrival William Harvey swore the Latin Oath of Matriculation at the Old Schools: 'The Advancement of Piety and good Learning, I will support', he vowed, 'So help me God, and the Holy Gospels of God.' He then entered his name in the Lists of Matriculation as 'Will. Harvie' and it was also inscribed in the Caius College Book, a weighty volume, bound in leather.* 'Wil. Harvey', the Latin entry reads, 'son of Thomas Harvey yeoman, from the town of Folkestone in the county of Kent, educated at Canterbury School, in his sixteenth year, has been admitted as *pensionarius minor* to the Scholars' mess on the last day of May 1593 . . . He pays for his entrance into the college three shillings and fourpence.'

Pensionarii minores were typically the sons of clergymen, professionals, merchants, yeomen or husbandmen; they could be either Bachelors of the Arts, bursaried scholars or commoners without financial support. Harvey entered as a commoner, but was elevated to the rank of scholar in the autumn of 1593, being awarded the Matthew Parker Scholarship, which carried a considerable stipend of £3 8d per annum. The scholarship was a medical one, the very first of its kind in England, so Harvey must already have shown some promise in the field. It was awarded only to former pupils of

---

*He was one of ten Caius students with the extremely common name 'Harvey' (variously spelt 'Harvie', 'Harvy', 'Harvye' or 'Hervey') to appear in that book over the period spanned by his lifetime; two of these students were also called 'William'.

the King's School, Canterbury, and to natives of Kent. The successful candidate had to prove himself to be 'able, learned, and worthy'; he also had to meet the bizarre criteria the college demanded of all its scholars—'that he be neither deformed, dumb, lame, maimed, mutilated, sick, invalid or Welsh'. Thomas Harvey may have known about the Matthew Parker Scholarship, and sent his eldest son to Caius with the command to secure it.

The scholarship placed Harvey in a more comfortable position, in financial terms, as well as for the additional social distance it placed between him and the 'sizars', classed below the *minores*. Sizars were officially poor young men who boarded, lodged and learned for free, paying their way through the menial tasks they performed for the fellows and the aristocratic students. The scholarship also placed Harvey a little closer to the gentlemen of the college, classified as *pensionarii majores*. Yet he was still separated, by some way, from that group which included the sons of noblemen (earls, lords and barons) and knights.

Gentlemen entered the university in ever increasing numbers as the sixteenth century progressed, largely because of Elizabeth's patronage of university men. Important positions in the church, state, professions, and even at court, were offered by the queen to graduates; by the end of her reign over half the Members of Parliament had been to Oxford or Cambridge. Many *pensionarii minores* were outraged by the pervasive presence of gentlemen in universities that had originally been 'erected by their founders for poor men's sons, whose parents were not able to bring them up unto learning . . . Now they have least benefit of them, by reason the rich do encroach upon them.'

Student daily life was unvarying. Having risen sometime after four in the morning to the sound of the college bell, Harvey, along with all 'of the fellows, scholars and students, who [had] not reached their fortieth year' prepared himself for chapel, where morning prayers and divine service commenced at five. Failure to appear was punished by a fine of at least twopence. Harvey's clerical gown had, according to the university statutes, to be 'decently' and 'respectably' presented; over it he put a surplice. On his broad head Harvey fixed his 'scholastic and square' cap.

Inside the fourteenth-century college chapel every individual had a place assigned to him according to his scholarly status—the fellows in the higher stalls, the students in the lower. Within the student ranks, social status determined position. Any one refusing to 'give place' (while doffing their cap) to a superior, was punished with a beating; the statutes decreed that 'modesty suited to their rank shall be cultivated everywhere. Inferior ranks shall give way to superior, and treat them with proper respect'.

Morning service was in strict accordance with the liturgy of the Protestant English Church, established by Elizabeth. In 1558, the first year of her reign, she had 'inspected and purged our Universities, the chief fountains of learning' so that 'superstition [i.e. Catholicism] the ruin of all true religion, may be put to flight, and ignorance, entirely banished'. From that date too, anyone wishing to graduate from Oxford or Cambridge had to acknowledge Elizabeth as the head of the church. Religious conformity was especially important now that so many scions of the most powerful English families attended university.

After chapel, at precisely 6.10 a.m., Harvey's studies began, continuing until ten, with only a short break for bread and beer. At ten a bell summoned Harvey to dinner in hall, in Gonville Court, a wooden-beamed building fairly small by Cambridge standards. The students sat according to rank, the superior young men on tables nearer to the fire. Gentlemen had a separate table where they were waited on by their sizars. The more generous aristocrats gave their servants 'leave to eat' at their expense when they found themselves in 'distress'—a permanent state for many sizars, who often had to pawn their books, and even beg on the public highways. Gratefully receiving a few coins from his master the sizar would bow and bound across the hall to make a 'lamentable cry at the buttery-hatch, "Ho, Lancelot, a cue of bread and a cue of beer."'

While gentlemen ordered lavish meals, *pensionarii minores* such as Harvey shared a penny piece of beef between four, some 'porage' made of the broth of the beef, a little oatmeal and a small glass of beer. Harvey's scholarship covered the costs of tuition, lodging and board, but permitted him to purchase food only of the most basic kind. After lunch, students might take a brisk postprandial walk in the city or the surrounding countryside. A restless country boy, Harvey must have loved to tramp the marshlands around Cambridge, following the silver Cam and its tributaries, abundant in perch and pike, over bridges, into orchards, through the grazing grounds of horses, cows, pigs and boars, past fields full of sheep and goats.

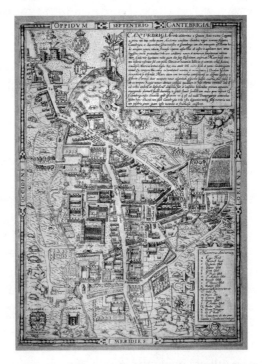

Richard Lynne's 1574 bird's-eye view of Cambridge. The city's historical centre resembles a heart, bordered by the River Cam and the Kinge's Ditch stream. The vein-like Cam, arriving from the south, passes King's and Clare, next to which we see 'Gunwell and Caius'.

In the afternoons, students studied until five, when they sat down to a scant dinner. Further reading took the young men up to compulsory evening service in chapel at seven, after which study continued until nine or ten. Students were then, according to one contemporary, 'fain to walk or run up and down half an hour, to get a heat in their feet' before going to bed.

For those who wearied of scholarly labour, there were temptations in town—'taverns, dicing, sword-playing, gaming, boxing-matches, skittle-playing, dancings, bear-fights, cock-fights and the like'; 'the like' including theatrical performances, and a plentiful supply of whores. The punishments for indulging in such recreations were so severe, however, that they would probably have deterred Harvey, who was, in any case, of a bookish and conformist temperament.

Yet nefarious activities went on, especially among gentlemen, who were allowed to purchase the privilege of transgressing many university decrees. A scholar such as Harvey always wore in public his clerical cloth gown, a cloak 'of black or sad [i.e dark] colour' and a cap of rough cloth (caps made of silk 'for the sake of softness or elegance' being forbidden); in private, a plain shirt and a hose made of simple material was compulsory. In contrast, gentlemen could parade the quads in velvet doublets and wear their hair long. They entertained each other in their rooms, too, and obtained permission to leave college for hours or even days at a time. 'Huntinge from morninge till nighte,' as one sizar described his masters' habits, 'they never studied nor gave themselves to their bookes, but [went] to schools of defence [i.e. fencing], to ye daun-cieing scolles, to stealle deer and connyes [rabbits] . . . to woinge of wenches.'

Such accomplishments were the traditional attributes of gentlemen, the ornaments of a courtier. University served as a finishing school, where they learned to ride, play tennis, master falconry. The well-born student who rarely looked into his books was a stock figure of fun in popular literature, even though the caricature was growing somewhat musty by the 1590s. 'Of all things', it was said, 'the young gentleman at University endures not to be mistaken for a scholar.' Gentlemen dismissed scholars as melancholy, pedantic and of low birth, utterly bereft of manners and civility; 'honest' they may have been, but they knew nothing of honour or decorum—true virtues because they were social rather than solitary.

Exposed to such attitudes, Harvey must have realized, during his first months at college, the acute difficulty of the mission his father had given him—the achievement of wealth and status in a world ruled by gentlemen. Three conventional strategies were now open to him in his bid to climb the social ladder.

He could study hard and attempt to stay on at Caius as a fellow, yet that would only constitute a partial social victory, as fellows were not gentlemen. Alternatively, Harvey could watch the aristocrats closely, and learn to imitate their ways. This had been the tactic of Christopher Marlowe, the son of a Canterbury shoemaker, who had excited comment in the quads by dressing in a flamboyant style. In one of his plays, Marlowe outlines the strategy, when a character advises his friend to:

> . . . cast the scholar off,
> And learn to court it like a gentleman.
> 'Tis not a black coat and a little band,
> A velvet-caped cloak faced before with serge . . .
> Or making low legs to a nobleman,
> Or looking downward with your eyelids close
> And saying 'Truly, an't may please Your Honour',
> Can get you any favour with great men.
> You must be proud, bold, pleasant, resolute . . .

Unlike his fellow Kentishman, however, Harvey lacked the requisite social graces, as well as the looks and the audacity, to carry off the scheme.

There was a third path, however, opened by Elizabeth's patronage of university men. A degree could be used as a passport to one of the professions and, thereafter, might facilitate access to the court. Nicholas Bacon, the son of a yeoman, and father of the philosopher Francis Bacon, considered himself to be 'half a gentleman' simply by virtue of his admission to Cambridge. On 'going down' from the university, he studied law at Gray's Inn, then became a barrister and eventually entered Parliament. He officially secured genteel status in 1558, the year in which Elizabeth appointed him Lord Keeper of the Seal. Soon afterwards she knighted him.

In electing to send his son to Cambridge, and in encouraging him to apply for the Parker Scholarship in medicine, Thomas Harvey probably hoped that William would tread a similar path. The choice of subject was a typically canny one: like the law, medicine offered the yeoman a clearly defined, albeit arduous, route to the professions and so (in many cases) on to gentlemanly status; respected medical men also tended on the nobility and their services were required at court. William had obediently concurred with his father's choice of subject and career; he may even have had some influence in the decision himself. A friend recalled that 'he thought again and again how he could raise himself effectively from the ground and place his head among the stars, and, at last, there settled in his mind the wish to embrace medicine'.

3. Cambridge studies II (c.1593–1599): 'Devoting himself assiduously to his studies'

ARVEY TOOK THE daily eighteen-hour grind in his short, rapid stride, racing to the end of each day's intellectual journey with the same alacrity with which he dashed across the college lawns. The undergraduate syllabus was based on the medieval division of the 'seven liberal arts' into the *trivium* (the 'three ways'), of rhetoric, ethics and logic, and the *quadrivium* (the 'four ways', or mathematical arts) of music, arithmetic, astronomy and geometry.

Rhetoric meant the study of Latin language and literature, with a little Greek and some Hebrew. It taught Harvey, in the words of the statutes, 'the nature of men's passions and affections', 'how to raise and move them' through words, and 'how to allay, quiet and change them'. Harvey had been prepared for the rigours of Cambridge rhetoric by his tutors at King's, Canterbury. By his fourth year at the grammar school, he knew how to inflect every noun and verb in Latin, and was 'practised in poetic tales, the familiar letters of learned men'. In his final year, he had mastered the art of varying his 'speech to every mood' and context. At Cambridge Harvey was urged to keep a commonplace book in order to gather there 'phrases and idioms' from poets, philosophers and historians. Their 'choice and witty sayings' would garnish his own discourse with a 'copiousness of word and good expressions, and also raise [his] fancy to a poetic strain'.

Harvey later told a medical colleague that, at Cambridge, he had 'drunk deep in poetry', which he revered as 'the purest and richest spring of all'. He was never happier than when busying himself, in his phrase, 'with the inner rites of Phoebus Apollo'. The god of his idolatry was the Roman poet, Virgil. Harvey was especially drawn to the *Eclogues* and the *Georgics* in which Virgil, a Mantuan yeoman's son, celebrates the beauties and virtues of the country life. The Kentishman read these poems in a state of rapture; coming to a more than usually magnificent passage he would throw the volume across the room with the exclamation 'He hath a devil!' Harvey would frequently quote Virgil, along with countless other classical authors, in his later writings on anatomy and physiology, which are themselves fine literary productions and models of rhetoric.

Harvey was drawn to philosophy too. The ethics course led Harvey through the problems, morals and politics of the fourth-century BC Greek philosopher Aristotle, with occasional detours to Pliny and Plato. During it, he was taught that the good life consisted of virtuous activity in the world, conducted under the dictates of reason. Logic, on the other hand, was 'the art of directing the mind in the acquisition of knowledge'; it taught Harvey the definition, naming and classification of things. Here again, the master was Aristotle, who dominated the landscape of the Renaissance imagination, with his famous 'four cause' method of classification. The 'material cause' related to the substance an object was made of (i.e. a chair is made of wood); the 'efficient cause' focused on its action, and the agency by which its movement was brought about (i.e. a football moves because it is kicked); the 'final cause' was its ultimate purpose (i.e. an acorn grows because it wants to be a tree); its 'formal cause' related to the type of thing it was (i.e. Elizabeth was a woman.)

Having classified an entity using the four causes, Harvey was then taught to build up propositions concerning it, by means of a syllogism. A syllogism begins with a universal major premise, is followed by a minor premise, and ends with a conclusion:

> All men are mortal.
> Socrates was a man.
> Therefore Socrates was mortal.

Harvey learned how to move his thoughts in accordance with these leaps of logic. He was taught that only conclusions reached via syllogisms had philosophical validity, just as objects could only exist in intellectual terms if their four causes were fully explained.

The *quadrivium* introduced Harvey to music, arithmetic, geometry and astronomy, and, in the process, to the principles of metaphysics, physics and mathematics. Metaphysics focused on 'being' and universal principles; physics concentrated on 'the principles of objects in motion', and investigated their qualitative aspects. Some branches of mathematics, such as arithmetic, concerned quantity and measurement instead; as a result, mathematics was often, as one student noted, looked down upon and hardly considered to be an '*Academical* study, but rather Mechanical; as the business of *Traders, Merchants, Seamen.*'

It was the duty of Harvey's tutor George Estey to oversee his studies. Conscientious tutors devised detailed programmes for their charges, yet many students complained of having 'none to direct [them], in what books to read, or what to seek, or in which method to proceed'. Estey may have left the intensely independent Harvey to his own devices.

University lectures at the Old Schools were compulsory, absence being punished with a twopenny fine. Usually beginning at 7 a.m., they lasted an hour. The gowned and capped students were required to remain 'quiet and attentive', but there was often a low murmur of noise and fidgeting in the wooden benches, especially in winter, as the students endeavoured to keep warm, and awake, in what was essentially an unheated barn. The lecturer typically took a passage from a classical author, 'glossed' it by elucidating linguistic or philosophical obscurities, then discussed the various commentaries it had inspired over the centuries. Students took verbatim notes—no easy task on the coldest days, with their hands frozen stiff.

Harvey played a more active role when it came to the 'declamation', a species of essay the student read out to his tutor. A declamation could also be public, performed in the Old Schools in front of university dignitaries. Harvey would be given a question to consider— 'Is spring the pleasantest season of the year?', 'Was Homer's Penelope faithful?'—and instructed to discuss it in 'perspicuous, smooth, plaine, vivid, masculine' Latin, embellishing his oration with illustrations and quotations from the classical authors.

A more argumentative and forceful style was required for the academic 'disputation'—a duel of words between a student who defended a thesis and several adversaries who offered objections to it, performed either in college or publicly at the Old Schools. Harvey had to dispute at least twice in public (once as defendant, once as opponent) before taking his Bachelor degree.

Public disputations began with a procession—the various disputants, accompanied by their tutors, walking solemnly from their colleges to form a line in front of the Old Schools. Harvey, leaving the Gate of Humility, made his slow progress southwards through the High Street, taking the first right down University Street and so under the arch of the Schools. The participants were then led into a vast hall inside the Old Schools by esquire bedells, dressed in tall hats and gowns.

As Harvey took his place at his designated stall the bell of the Old Schools rang one o'clock, then the bedell declared '*Bona nova, Bona nova*' ('Good news, good news'—the entire affair being conducted in Latin). The vice chancellor sat down in his chair as Harvey, if cast in the defending role, 'made curtsy' to him (in three customary bows), as well as to his various opponents, saying '*Gratias ago vobis*' (Thank you) to each. The vice chancellor recited a prayer and made a short speech, before the moderator (always a don) announced to 'their highnesses' the theses that would be disputed. The theses were posted on the door of the Old Schools at least eight days before the disputation to give the participants time to prepare. These might be anything from 'The production of the rational soul involves a new creation', to 'The threat of punishment is a sufficient deterrent of crime', all seven of the 'liberal arts' providing topics for discussion. The discussion of controversial political and religious subjects was, however, expressly forbidden under the Elizabethan statutes.

The moderator, having made his own general comment on the theses, asked the defending student's tutor to make a speech on behalf of his charge; Estey spoke for Harvey. Meanwhile the bedell presented to the vice chancellor some Latin verses Harvey had composed on the theme of the theses, which served as an elegant introduction to the debate. Estey proceeded to raise potential objections to the theses—straw men that Harvey could dispatch easily, as a means of limbering up for the duel proper.

The first opponent (who had to be a member of a different college) then attacked one thesis, attempting to force the defendant into logical and rhetorical dead ends. While the participants should not, according to the moderator, become too 'hot & fiery & fierce', neither should they recite their arguments mechanically, but speak always with vigour and imagination. Colourful exclamations reverberated around the walls and ceiling of the Old Schools as the disputants had at each other. 'I progress with my argument thus' came the thrust; 'You are not progressing, but merely shifting your ground', the clever parry. '*Tuo gladio jugulabo!*' cried the student who sensed victory— 'Now I will slit your throat with your own rhetorical sword.'

For three hours the argument twisted and turned in the dank air, accompanied by the encouragement and applause of the audience. If the speeches became convoluted the moderators disentangled the rhetorical and logical knots; they also cut short tedious lines of enquiry. A disputation was also intended as entertainment, with local nobles, dignitaries and even the queen herself sometimes attending. At the end of the proceedings the vice chancellor would declare as winner either the defendant or the challengers. The victor would be cheered as enthusiastically as a triumphant fencer after a match, before being led out of the Old Schools in procession.

Circular disputations, held at college in chapel or hall, were less formal affairs, with a number of defendants and opponents standing in a circle, each student taking an argument up where his predecessor's voice trailed off. Yet they could be equally heated. Many gentlemen objected to the discord and violence disputations inspired. In their view, the exercise encouraged litigiousness, and turned young men into 'excellent wranglers—which art, though it may be tolerable in a mercenary lawyer' was hardly the attribute of a 'sober and well-governed gentleman', whose aim was always to promote social harmony.

Harvey, however, stood on the side of the academic authorities, who believed that 'disputations lead not only to knowledge of the truth, but also to promptitude, and to boldness in scholars'. He relished the rhetorical swordplay, becoming famous in later life, and perhaps even among his Cambridge peers, as a 'wrangler' of genius.

Harvey completed his arts course in the customary four years, graduating in 1597. He more than merited his degree. With an intellect 'not to be held bound by the laws of a single discipline' he took, a friend said, 'the whole of Nature', and the entire intellectual universe, 'as his province', reading beyond the bounds of the course.

From 1597 Harvey focused much of his attention on medicine, one of the 'sciences'* he was now at liberty to study. The subject

* The word 'science', meant 'study' in its broadest sense, and only acquired its modern signification of knowledge derived through experimentation and observation in the first half of the nineteenth century.

was in its infancy at Cambridge, the teaching conservative and second rate by continental standards. Still, Harvey was at the best college to study it. A physician and scholar of international renown, John Caius had established two medical college fellowships; he had also stipulated that the fellows organize regular medical disputations and an annual dissection in college. Because of a paucity of suitable corpses or sufficiently skilled practitioners, this statute was, however, largely ignored.

To 'raise himself effectively from the ground' and place 'his head among the stars' Harvey needed to master more medical knowledge than Cambridge had to offer. He appears to have embarked on an intense and sustained course of 'private' reading—private meaning individual rather than solitary. Only gentlemen could afford to live alone in college, their spacious and lavishly furnished rooms costing over a pound a year in rent. Harvey had to share a spartan room with his tutor and as many as three other students. The students studied and slept in an attic known as the cockloft, which was reached by a ladder from the tutor's room below. In this tiny eyrie, the student had his own narrow hard bed and wooden study cubicle. Casements gave him a partial view of the quad, but offered no glass protection from the wind or the damp air that rose from the fens around Cambridge. Fireless, the loft was scarcely habitable in winter, when the student's ink would freeze in its well.

The alternative was to read in the college library, a long white medieval room, with five windows on either side and a large window at the end. Walking through it, Harvey passed a series of wooden bays with lecterns, beneath which numerous chained leather volumes were shelved. Entering a bay, Harvey bent down to pick up a heavy folio volume, then placed it on the lectern in front of him; remaining standing he opened it, and began to read. The library was the quietest and one of the brightest rooms in the college. Yet, as the day waned, the gloom spread along with the cold, there being neither artificial lighting nor heating. Harvey, hunched over his book in the dwindling light, peering down ever more closely at the printed or handwritten words, might have struck any gentleman present as the very emblem of the book-fool.

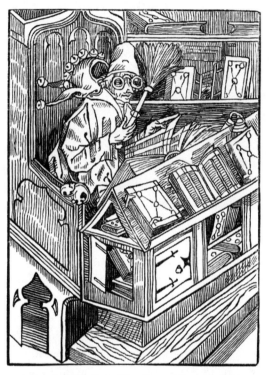

A 'book-fool' from *The Ship of Fools* (1509).

Yet though Harvey may often have been seen reading at Cambridge, he was by no means a book-fool. He despised 'bookish' study divorced from experience, and frequently criticized pedants. It is easy to imagine him laughing at, and agreeing with, Michel de Montaigne's (1533–1592) famous contemporary caricature of the block-headed book-fool. 'When I ask him what he knows', Montaigne remarked, 'he asks me for a book in order to point it out to me, and wouldn't tell me that he has an itchy backside unless he goes immediately and studies in his lexicon what is itchy and what backside.'

Harvey gained a scholarly reputation among Caius students by 'devoting himself assiduously to his studies'. Overzealous students often set peers gossiping, and gentlemen laughing in scorn. It was rumoured of one young man that he 'went not out of the College gates in a good while, nor (I think) out of his Chamber, but was in his slip shoes, and wore out his gowne and cloathes on the bord and benches of his chamber, but profited in knowledge exceedingly'. No such anecdotes of Harvey survive, however, his affable nature perhaps tempering his image as a 'gown-man'.

There may have been a rule at Caius, as there was in the University Library, 'that none tarry at one booke above one hour'. In that case, Harvey would have had to read hard, and with fero-cious speed and concentration—something that came easily, no doubt, to the alert and eager young man. Students were advised to accompany their reading with 'perpetual meditations, repetitions, recapitulations, reiterations' and 'deepe imprinting in ye memory'.

Harvey read the works of Galen with wrapt attention. His well-thumbed copy of the Greek physician's *Miscellaneous Writings* (studied during a later period of his life and one of the few books from his library to have survived) attests to the concentration he lavished on the author. Students were encouraged to highlight difficult phrases, or matters of special observation in books—to literally mark an author's words. 'Doe it', they were instructed, 'with little lines under them, or above them . . . to the end that you may oftimes reade over these, until you be perfect in them.' They were also urged to 'gloss' obscure sentences, writing out definitions in the margin in simple Latin. On some pages of Harvey's Galen every sentence is underlined; on many pages he glosses a word or phrase from the text. He also made countless notes in the margins of the book, and some of his annotations are rather droll. At one point, Galen declares that learning is a superior attribute to social rank, being internal, rather than external to man. As an illustration of this idea Harvey scribbled the words 'wooden leggs' in the margin, vividly conjuring up the image of a man attempting to raise his status by 'external' means—i.e. walking on stilts. When he reached the end of the book, Harvey followed scholarly etiquette, by compiling a list of subjects of interest, as a sort of personalized index, for easy reference at a later date.

The college library was well stocked with Galen's works, John Caius having bequeathed many of the Greek's writings to the college. Caius had himself edited a Greek edition of Galen's *Anatomical Procedures* during his spell as a student, and tutor, at the University of Padua in the 1540s. Exemplary Renaissance humanist, and devoted disciple of Galen that he was, Caius aimed to restore the pristine Greek original, the text having been corrupted over the centuries. It was a Herculean labour, but also a labour of love for Caius, who believed Galen to be virtually infallible. Caius' edition, along with other Galenic texts in the college library, shrouded the Greek physician in an aura of what Harvey called 'omnipotence'.

As he stood in Caius library, Harvey read Galen's works with reverence and concentration, his beady eyes scouring them for passages of particular interest. He would transcribe these in his commonplace book, where he stored all the 'best things out of an author', for future use in declamations and at disputations. Later on, after a long day's reading, when the light had faded, Harvey closed up the volumes he had been studying, set them back in their places, and walked out of the valley of the shadow of books.

❧ Essay 1 ☙

Galen, Mondino, and Vesalius:
A brief history of anatomy

AFTER EXTENSIVE STUDY and travel, Galen (c. AD 130–200) eventually settled in Imperial Rome. Endlessly curious about human anatomy and physiology, the physician dissected hundreds of living and dead animals in a bid to map the human body. The dissection of human corpses had been common in Alexandria in the fourth and third centuries BC, but it was forbidden by law throughout the Roman Empire, as the Romans venerated the dead and had a superstitious fear of cadavers. Galen did not regard this decree as a serious impediment to his investigations, holding the orthodox view that pigs and primates had fundamentally the same anatomy as man, however distinct man was from them in spiritual and intellectual terms.

A showman of genius, Galen often carried out his dissections in public, making a great splash among the Roman elite. He became physician to the gladiators, patching up their wounds between bouts in the Coliseum, and later doctor to the emperors. Galen's achievement was to systemize, elaborate and popularize the teachings of the school of Hippocrates, the Greek father of medicine, born in the fifth century BC. So comprehensive and coherent were Galen's Hippocratic theories that they gained almost universal acceptance and continued to hold intellectual sway right up to Harvey's time.

Galen held that there was an intimate connection between the structure, purpose and functioning of an organ. Each organ worked autonomously, attracting to itself whatever it needed in order to transform the various substances of the body. These substances moved slowly within the body, where they were consumed and replaced.

The lungs produced phlegm, the gall bladder yellow bile (choler), black bile (melancholy) came from the spleen, and blood from the liver. These substances constituted the body's four basic humours. In *On the Temperaments*, Galen argued that the predominance of a particular humour determined a man's temperament or 'complexion', which could be either melancholic, phlegmatic, sanguine or choleric. Reading that book, or Galen's *Art of Physic*, Harvey may have recognized his own character and physique in the Greek's description of the choleric man, for he was, according to his friends, a 'very Colerique . . . hott-head'. 'We call that man choleric', Galen wrote, 'in whose body heat and dryness abounds . . . Such persons are usually short of stature, and not fat . . . their skin rough and hot in feeling . . . the colour of their face is tawny or sunburnt; they have beards; they have little hollow hazel eyes . . . their pulse is swift and strong . . . they dream of fighting, quarrelling, fire . . . they are naturally quick-witted, bold, furious, hasty, eloquent, courageous, stout-hearted creatures, not given to sleep much, but much given to jesting.' Along with these characteristics, the choleric type was thought to be ambitious, industrious, energetic, passionate, independent, forthright and overbearing—all attributes Harvey displayed.

According to Galen, a short-term excess or deficiency of a humour produced illness. This could be treated by decisive, localized, intervention—the cause of the disease often being diagnosed as a malfunction of the productive organ in question. Bloodletting in the affected area of the body was recommended. The regulation of diet was also important, as food could be acted upon by an organ to produce a certain humour. If the disease were wet and hot, such as fever, then dry and cold foods were prescribed. The key to health was maintaining the humours in a state of balance (*eucrasia*); *dycrasia*, imbalance, might in some cases even result in death.

At Cambridge, Harvey had to imprint these ideas on his memory. Galen formed the basis of the medical syllabus, and theses at disputations were often inspired by his theories and therapies; 'A humour is a quality' being a typical example, or 'A cold stomach is better for appetite than a warm one'. Harvey also learned many specific Galenic notions by rote in preparation for periodic interrogations by his tutor. 'Why doth a woman sometime conceive twins?' the tutor demanded; 'According unto Galen', the industrious student would answer, 'because there is more than one cel or receptacle of seed in the womb.' Galen had to be mastered in such detail partly because some of the students were destined to become physicians, and their treatments would be based upon his theories.

Harvey also studied Galen's theory of the function of the heart, an organ which played a crucial role in the distribution of humours and spirits within the body. Galen argued that there were two distinct and parallel vascular systems—the veins, originating in the liver, and the arteries, beginning at the heart. He derived this idea from his numerous dissections and vivisections of animals, during which he observed that the veins and arteries were utterly separate and also different—the arteries being much thicker, and having the innate capacity to pulsate. Blood moving around these systems was quite distinct too, the one being purple, the other red.

The first system, according to Galen, distributed *nutritive* blood which was created in the liver, the body's most important organ. The liver actively sucked chyle into itself from the stomach, which had produced that milky substance by digesting food. In the liver, chyle was concocted into viscous purple blood and imbued with the 'natural spirit' that animates all living things. From the liver the nutritive blood was distributed slowly through the veins (hence its other name 'venous blood') to the extremities of the body—both below and above the liver, and even back to the stomach, in order to replenish all the muscles and bones. A certain amount of blood entered the right side of the heart via the vena cava, some of it continued on its upward journey past the heart. In the veins the blood flowed backwards and forwards in slow motion, the organs 'attracting' blood to themselves and consuming it.

Galen's second blood system focused on the heart. When the right ventricle of the heart sucked venous blood into itself through the vena cava one of two things happened to it. Some of it travelled to the lungs via the vena arteriosa (known today as the pulmonary artery), its impurities being expelled through that organ by means of exhalation. The remainder moved to the left ventricle of the heart through pores in the muscular wall (or septum) that divided the heart's right and left ventricles. Here it was mixed with 'vital spirit' known as pneuma or 'divine breath', which entered the lungs as inhaled air, and travelled to the heart via the arteria venosa (now known as the pulmonary vein). The Greeks believed that pneuma represented the soul within the body, facilitating all thought and sensation, and allowing the movement of the muscles and limbs.

In the left side of the heart the mingled blood and pneuma were boiled in a process known as 'concoction'. This transformed the liquid into vivified arterial blood, changing its colour from dark purple to scarlet. When the arterial blood overflowed in the left side of the heart it was drawn into the aorta, which slowly distributed the liquid throughout the body, in an ebbing and flowing motion; some of this blood also returned to the lungs via the arteria venosa. The organs of the body consumed the arterial blood, with any surplus evaporating; the liquid could never dry up within the body because the liver produced it continuously. The 'vital' spirits engendered in the heart, along with the nutritive 'natural' spirits formed in the liver, were converted into 'animal' spirits in the brain, thereby making the human body animate, intelligent and spiritual.

For Galen the heart worked like a set of bellows, expanding to draw pneuma-filled air into itself from the lungs, then, in contracting, expelling impurities through them. The organ needed air for two reasons: it required pneuma, and it had to stay cool. The origin of all the body's 'innate heat', the heart worked like a furnace to concoct the blood. The heart was therefore intimately connected with the lungs, and functioned as part of the respiratory system. According to Galen, the heart did not regulate the blood's flow within the body; rather, it was determined by the attractive power of each organ, the pulsative force of the arteries, and the general ebb and flow of the humours within the body.

In the medieval period anatomists began dissecting human corpses, the Catholic Church having discontinued the Roman prohibition of the practice. The human body was, in its view, the high point of God's creation, a little world as 'wondrous' in its harmony and complexity as the universe itself. It was deemed eminently worthy of display at university anatomies, the first documented public dissection being conducted by Mondino de Luzzi (c.1270–1326) at the University of Bologna in 1315.

In 1316 Mondino penned his *Anathomia Corporis Humani* (*Anatomy of the Human Body*), which would remain the practical and theoretical handbook for anatomists for over 200 years. The volume begins with the overtly Christian declaration that man, being the summit of creation, is the worthiest subject of scholarly enquiry. Despite being based on the personal experience of cutting up countless human corpses, Mondino's volume reverently repeated the theories that Galen had derived, over 1,000 years previously, from his exclusive study of animal carcasses. Such was the Greek physician's eminence and appeal that the medieval anatomist aimed only to summarize him, any contradiction being tantamount to heresy. Mondino is indeed unlikely to have perceived any need to revise Galen, for when anatomists looked down at the open human corpse, they simply viewed what the master had taught them to see. Galen's theories continued to work their magic beyond the time of Leonardo da Vinci (1452–1519), whose famous anatomical drawings, though sketched from real cadaver models, are heavily influenced by the Greek physician's ideas.

Yet challenges to Galen's dominion were not long in coming. With the publication of countless scholarly published editions of Galen's works (following the advent of the printing press in the fifteenth century), along with a profusion of public anatomies, it became far easier for anatomists to test Galen's specific theories directly against the dissected human corpse.

The Belgian anatomist Andreas Vesalius (1514–64) was the supreme dissector of the age. Having edited several of Galen's texts, he also knew the Greek's oeuvre by heart. After completing his doctorate in medicine at the University of Padua, the twenty-three-year-old prodigy was offered the chair of surgery and anatomy there. From that eminent position (and also as anatomist at the nearby University of Bologna), he gave his medical students revolutionary courses in anatomy.

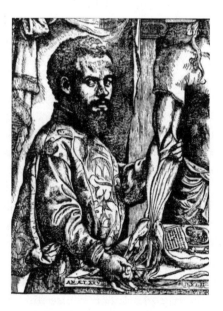

In this 1543 portrait Vesalius displays the muscles in the forearm of a female corpse. On the table there is an anatomical knife and a pen, as though the Belgian wishes to advertise his ability with both instruments.

Traditionally an anatomical performance involved three pro-tagonists. The professor played the part of the *lector*, reading out passages from a textbook such as Mondino's *Anathomia*, and gener-ally remaining seated throughout the dissection. An *ostensor*, or demonstrator (one of the professor's assistants), taking his cue from the *lector*, would show the *sector* (the other assistant, usually a lecturer of surgery or a local barber) which sections of the body were to be dissected. After the *sector* had opened up the body with a knife, the *ostensor* would proceed to indicate to the audience, with a rod, the organs and parts to which the *lector* referred in his recitation. The textbook was at the centre of this performance, and the body a sort of three-dimensional illustration.

At the University of Bologna the convention had been altered by Vesalius' time. The professor delivered an anatomical lecture in the hall, which was followed by a dissection in a separate chamber, performed by an *ostensor*-cum-*sector*, and intended to illustrate and explicate the professor's address. When Vesalius was called upon to perform this latter role, he deliberately exceeded his remit. Sometimes he would ignore the professor's lecture, focusing on issues of greater interest to himself; at others he would flatly contradict the professor, and an argument would erupt between the pair.

Entrusted on other occasions with the task of organizing demonstra-tions himself, this star of the anatomy theatre, eager for attention and critical of those 'fashionable doctors' who 'despised the work of the hand', chose to combine the three roles of *lector*, *ostensor* and *sector*. As he cut away, the Belgian summarized rather than read from ana-tomical authorities, his hands being much too occupied to hold a book.

Students were drawn to the content as well as the energy of Vesalius' performances. He offered these aspiring physicians and surgeons exactly the type of anatomy course they craved, providing a complete education in surgery and dissection, a comprehensive discussion of the entire human body, and an introduction to the various diseases that the organs were heir to. Vesalius always

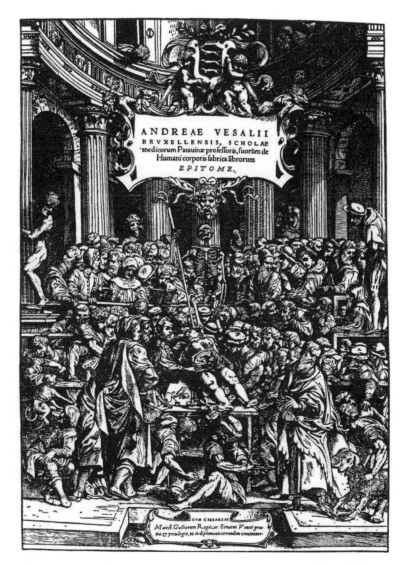

The title page of an *Epitome* of Vesalius' *De humani corporis fabrica* (*On the Structure of the Human Body*) (1543). This representation of Vesalius dissecting a female corpse is symbolic: the skeleton emphasizes the religious aspect of anatomy, the figures from the classical world underline Vesalius' eminence. An anatomical textbook is conspicuous by its absence.

encouraged his audience to 'see for themselves' (the original meaning of the word *autopsia*, or autopsy). He allowed spectators to stand right next to the corpse, and even to touch it. 'I took the lung in my hands', one of his students recorded, 'and it was very light like a sponge. There was a great quantity of blood in it.'

Vesalius' innovative style of anatomy* concentrated on the particular details of the dissected body. This made close comparisons between orthodox theory and the dissected human cadaver virtually inevitable. It took a man of Vesalius' genius and audacity, however, to identify and announce the discrepancies between them. In the course of his dissections, Vesalius discovered some 200 'errors' in Galen, which he blithely broadcast to his wonderstruck students, offering the human body as evidence. 'Even if what I say is not Galen's opinion,' he would declare, 'we shall demonstrate here, with this body, that it is in fact so. Everyone will be able to see it for himself'.

So plentiful were the mistakes Vesalius discerned that he eventually came to the conclusion that Galen must have dissected animal cadavers rather than human corpses. This was something previous anatomists had failed to grasp, being unaware of the Roman prohibition on human anatomies. Even if one of Vesalius' predecessors had intuited it, it is hard to believe they would have dared to proclaim it to the world. When Vesalius announced his discovery (in the 'corrected' editions of Galen's texts he published between 1539 and 1542) he was ignored or ridiculed by most professors, who still regarded Galen as 'most perfect and complete'. Their negative response may help explain why Vesalius was tentative in his criticisms of Galen in his 1543 anatomical manual, *De humani corporis fabrica*.

The Belgian had, for example, left his student audiences in little doubt of his view that there were no pores in the septum of the

---

*'Anatomy' is often used here as a synonym for 'dissection'; the word derives from the Greek *anatemnein*, 'to cut up'.

heart, yet when he discussed the issue in the *Fabrica* he was hesitant and evasive. As no pores 'perceptible to the senses' allow blood to move from the right to the left ventricle, 'we are', he equivocated, 'greatly forced to wonder at the skill of the Artificer of all things by which the blood sweats through the passages that are invisible to sight'.

In the second edition of the *Fabrica* (1555) Vesalius was a little bolder. 'In considering the structure of the heart', he remarked, 'I have brought my words for the most part into agreement with the teachings of Galen: not because I thought that these were on every point in harmony with the truth, but because I still distrust myself . . . But the septum of the heart is as thick, dense, and compact as the rest of the heart. I do not therefore know, in what way even the smallest particle can be transferred [through it].'

Harvey could have read Vesalius' famous words in Cambridge University Library's copy of the 1555 edition. Caius library may also have boasted a first or second edition. John Caius had a particular interest in Vesalius, having been friends with the Belgian during his student days in Italy. The two men had shared rooms in Padua, where they worked together on preparing editions of Galen's writings. Given the Englishman's reverence for Galen, and Vesalius' acute understanding of the Greek's limitations, they made for a volatile editorial partnership. One day, when going through a text, Vesalius came across what he believed to be an obvious interpolation, and deleted the line. Caius, however, was convinced of its authenticity, and demanded the line be restored. A scholarly stand-off ensued, and was never resolved, the peevish pair eventually going their separate ways. Nevertheless Caius' admiration for Vesalius seems to have remained undimmed by their argument, and by their divergence over Galen's theories. He wrote an introductory study of the *Fabrica* which he deposited in the college library, where Harvey could have taken it from the shelves.

4. Paduan studies I (1599–c.1600): 'Fair Padua, nursery of the arts'

ON 4 JULY 1599 Harvey left Caius for the long summer vacation. Some months later Harvey asked the college for permission to remain absent from the university beyond the beginning of the next term. He was suffering, he said, from a serious illness and required time and isolation to recover fully, doubtless at his family home in Kent. The illness may have been malaria, as Harvey would later complain of having been afflicted, at some point in his youth, by the 'ague' and by a 'tumour' on the liver—two symptoms of the disease. Harvey eventually returned to Caius on 27 October, but by then he had evidently made up his mind to leave university for good.

Harvey's illness may have been a factor in his decision to 'go down' from Cambridge, malaria and other serious diseases being pervasive in the damp Fenlands. Yet it is more likely that he chose to leave before completing his medical degree for academic reasons. The statutes of Caius permitted students of medicine to finish their studies on the Continent, in Montpellier, Bologna or Padua, which boasted far more prestigious schools of medicine than Cambridge. Any Englishman wishing to place 'his head among the stars' of learning, and who aimed at raising himself from the ground through professional success as a physician, could not afford to linger on his intellectually infertile native ground.

No doubt after consulting his father, who must have felt confident enough in his son's abilities to fund his further studies and travels, Harvey selected Padua University. His choice may have been influenced by an exposure to the works of Vesalius, who had taught in the Italian city; the famous modern anatomical school the Belgian had founded at the University was a Mecca for medical students throughout Europe. Another consideration may have been that Padua was John Caius' alma mater.

On 30 October Harvey left Caius. We do not know if he made his exit via the Gate of Honour, but he had certainly earned the right to do so, having taken his arts degree back in 1597. He was worthy of the honour too, in a broader sense, as few Caius students could have stuck more unswervingly to the path of assiduous study, humility, virtue and wisdom symbolized in the college's layout, than William Harvey.

The twenty-two-year-old embarked on his journey to Italy in the spring of 1600, travelling the short distance from Folkestone to the port of Dover. When Harvey showed his pass, the governor singled him out from a party about to board the boat for Calais. 'You must not go', the governor said, 'but must be kept prisoner.' Harvey desired to know for what reason he was detained. 'Well,' replied the governor, 'it is my Will to have it so.'

The packet boat on which Harvey should have travelled hoisted sail in the evening, leaving behind a smouldering Kentishman on the shore, where he was forced to spend the night. He regarded all such delays as 'unjust', 'barbarous' and 'tirannous'; he was a young man in a hurry ever 'greedy to be gone'. Any officials who obstructed him were 'most base and evel people', incapable of dealing 'playnly and rowndly'.

During the early hours of the next day a terrible storm ensued and the packet boat capsized. All of the passengers (among them many of Harvey's acquaintances) were drowned. When the tragic news reached Dover the doctor sought out the governor to ask him why he alone of the company had been detained and thereby saved. After all, Harvey was 'unknown to the Governor, both by Name and Face'. 'Two nights previously', the governor said, 'I saw a perfect Vision in a Dream of Doctor Harvey, who came to pass over to Calais; and I was given a warning to stop you.'

Harvey often told this story to his acquaintances, ascribing his good fortune to God's providence. Yet as well as illustrating his piety, the tale—and Harvey's fondness for telling it—also suggest a man who believed that he had been marked out for greatness.

Apart from the desire to complete his medical studies abroad, Harvey 'thought', according to a friend, 'that he should [also] travel . . . in the hope of acquiring thereby . . . teaching and wisdom . . . after the manner of the ancient philosophers (as they say about Plato and Pythagoras)'. Travel was moreover regarded as a social education for any young man aspiring to genteel status. To these ends, Harvey spent a few months visiting France and Germany before journeying down to Padua, having been supplied with the necessary funds by his father.

Along with money, Thomas probably furnished his eldest son with advice. Italy was notorious as the great continental market for gambling, drinking and whoring; the place where, it was popularly believed, an Englishman learned 'the art of atheism (synonymous, for the Elizabethans, with Catholicism), of epicurizing, of poisoning'; he became proud in demeanour, prolix and pretentious in speech, depraved in morals, and above all grasping, calculating and two-faced. The strict yeoman patriarch had no desire to see Harvey return to him as an *inglese italianizzato* (Italianized Englishman).

Yet Thomas would also have known that Italy was the cradle of the new humanistic learning. Ever since the thirteenth century, its scholars and artists laboured to restore, emulate, and even to surpass the philosophical wisdom and cultural achievements of the classical world (that wisdom having been locked up in so many ancient texts that had been recently recovered, and shorn of their interpolations). In *The Taming of the Shrew*, first performed in the 1590s, Lucentio enters Padua for the first time in a state of euphoria, having finally satisfied his great desire 'To see fair Padua, nursery of the arts'. He resolves to 'plunge him in the deep' philosophical waters, 'And with satiety . . . quench his thirst.'

Padua was the intellectual capital of the Venetian Republic and one of the jewels of north-east Italy. Padua's historical heart, situated on the most westerly of the three tiny islands that comprised it, beat very quickly. Every day hundreds of tradesmen and farmers flooded the city's vast market squares and jostled with noblemen and students in the labyrinthine streets. The clothes of the nobility must have dazzled Harvey with their colourful splendour: the men wrapped themselves up in long blue or red silk mantles; the women carried jewel-encrusted gloves and fans, and dyed their hair blonde, after the Venetian fashion. They were paraded around the piazzas in sedan chairs, by liveried servants, as though they were living works of art.

Attire denoted rank and profession. Students, immediately recognizable by their black gowns, were placed within the social hierarchy according to the status of their families. Whenever representatives of different classes met on the pavement, by law the social inferior was obliged to step down into the road. Stepping down was a serious business, in part because it was such a dirty one. Goats and cows ate and defecated in the highways, and citizens diluted their excrement by micturating everywhere, especially near the government buildings.

Padua University was known locally as 'Il Bo' (the Ox), having been built on the site of a famous fifteenth-century inn whose sign was an ox's head. The transformation of the inn, and surrounding buildings, into the magnificent Palazzo del Bo was the work of a century; the finishing touches were still being put to the facade in Harvey's time.

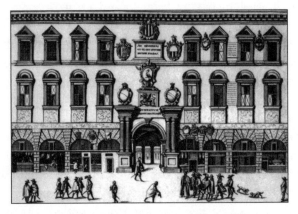

The facade of the Palazzo del Bo *c*. 1600.

Where the gates of Caius symbolized moral qualities, the entrance of the Bo was an eloquent emblem of temporal power. Students walking beneath the arch were watched closely by the animal perched on top of it—the lion of St Mark, symbol of the Venetian Republic's century-long hegemony over Padua. The winged lion had reason to be watchful as the university was the alma mater of the sons of those Venetian aristocrats whose names were written in the city's famous golden book. The future rulers of Venice had to be protected from harm, as well as from any form of political radicalism that might disturb the legendary harmony of La Serenissima, the 'most serene' Republic of Venice.

Venetian sovereignty gave the university great freedom in religious matters. A bitter rival of Rome, the republic ensured that the Vatican had limited influence over the institution, which was, in consequence, extremely tolerant of non-Catholics. It had offered a safe haven to English Protestants during the turbulent reign of 'Bloody' Mary, and attracted Protestants and Jews from Northern Europe. Among its 1,500 members there were it was said 'more students of forraine and remote nations then in any one University of Christendome'.

Students were organized into their various 'Nations', each of which had a representative *consiliarius* (councillor). This was a position of some influence in a university run entirely by the students. University statutes had to conform to the broader laws of the republic, yet within those limits students could determine the daily working of the institution, devising their own courses, selecting and paying the professors. The choice of tutors was often inspired: Vesalius had taught there, and Galileo Galilei was occupying the chair of mathematics when Harvey arrived.

Soon after his arrival, in the summer of 1600, Harvey paid a mandatory visit to the councillor of the English Nation. Entering the main gate of the Bo, he passed into the cool shade and calming quiet of the recently built sand-coloured courtyard, which had a double loggia held up by Doric and Ionic columns.

The English councillor organized Harvey's matriculation, and advised the freshman where to find lodgings. On his limited budget, Harvey could either reside with a professor such as Galileo, who had turned his home into a student hostel, or share a large room with another student, just as John Caius had done with Vesalius. Either way, his room would have been in one of the tall narrow buildings of the historical centre; cramped, dark and fireless, its windows were covered only with linen sheets. Harvey's landlord provided board along with lodging. The food was probably of limited quality by the luxurious standards of the Veneto, but the variety and plenty of the cheap fruit and vegetables, available all year round, made many simple meals seem like banquets to English students.

By law, Harvey's landlord had to ensure that his tenant did not stash firearms in his rooms; he was, however, permitted to keep a sword. Officially sported only on ceremonial occasions, and with express permission from the university and the civic authorities, swords were in fact worn on a daily basis, and with good reason. Bandits patrolled the vaulted city arcades after sundown, where they preyed upon drunken students, robbing them of their money and clothes.

The students were, however, usually far more comfortable in the role of aggressor than that of victim. There are numerous reports of their rampaging through the city. One more than usually boisterous spree took place in Harvey's time, when some students ransacked the shops of the historical centre, then broke into two monasteries. There they pummelled the monks and set all their chickens free. Immediately after the attack the monks and the shopkeepers joined forces in the public squares, drumming up reinforcements with the chant 'Kill, kill, kill all the students!'

The various student nations often challenged each other to armed combat. One evening during this period, the Italians were out scouring the city for their hated enemies the French, when they happened upon some Germans, whom they mistook for their rivals. The Italians proceeded to attack the unsuspecting party with swords, spears and stones. After a few seconds, they realized their error, but decided to continue the onslaught on the grounds that the Germans were almost as odious as the French. The Italian students also frequently fought among themselves—the Bresciani against the Trentini, the Veronesi against the Bergamaschi, the Genoese often challenging the Venetians, their old enemy in numerous wars of the medieval period.

It is not known whether Harvey participated in these violent delights, but it is possible. It certainly seems likely that it was at Padua that the proud Englishman acquired his habit of wearing a dagger. Whenever roused to anger, the 'very cholerique' Harvey would, in later life, finger the pommel of the dagger, and 'be apt to draw it out . . . upon every slight occasion'. The streets of Padua offered daily occasions for him to display such bravado, and to learn how to handle his weapon of choice; there provocative insults— '*Ma, non vorrete mica attaccar briga?*' ('Do you quarrel sir?')—led quickly to the drawing of swords, followed by futile attempts to keep the peace—'*Fermi, insensati, fermi! Giù le spade! Andate in pace, O!*' ('Put down your swords. Part, fools! Go in peace.')

Walking through the courtyard of the Bo, Harvey heard Flemish, Polish, Russian, Spanish, Magyar and Dutch, as well as the various

Italian dialects. Yet along with the cosmopolitan accents and colours of this brave new world, there were also familiar shades and sounds. The English Nation was dominated by gentlemen who came to Padua to perfect the aristocratic arts of dancing, fencing, hunting and music, and to acquire that effortless *sprezzatura* for which Italians were famous. As at Cambridge, whenever an English gentleman approached on the pavement, Harvey halted, bowed low, and stepped down into the dung of the street.

English students such as Harvey, hailing from the lower classes, attended Padua University with an eye to a career back home, in the law, the church or the medical establishment. Yet Harvey also aimed higher than membership of a professional elite, expressing to friends the hope of becoming a 'second Aesculapius' (the Roman god of medicine). He doubtless wished to emulate those English alumni of Padua who had won immortal renown for their intellectual achievements. Along with Caius, there was the physician Thomas Linacre, who also achieved fame as the editor of Galenic texts. These two men had been among the first scholars to import Italian human-istic studies into England.

As a statement of intent, only a few months after his arrival, Harvey put himself forward for the vacant position of councillor of the English Nation. His election campaign was a success. Although the opposition may have been limited, Harvey's triumph testifies to his ambition and confidence, especially as aristocrats had often occupied the position previously.

In the autumn of 1600, Harvey removed his students' gown and replaced it with a darker, more capacious mantle, the symbol of his newly acquired councillor status. In this garb, which must have threat-ened to engulf his tiny frame, he witnessed the matriculations and graduations of English students, fought their corner in the university senate, and cast their vote in the election of the all-important rector.

Councillors had to provide the university with a copy of their stemma, or coat of arms, to be emblazoned on the walls and vaults of the courtyard. Not being a gentleman, Harvey had no arms, so he set about designing his own elaborate symbol. Against a red background, a white right arm, issuing from the right, holds a white candle with a golden flame. Around the candle two green entwined serpents lean towards the fire.

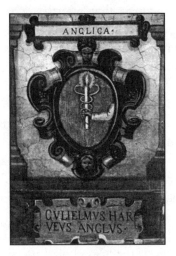

Harvey's stemma.

The serpents recalled Aesculapius, whose traditional symbol was a snake coiled around a staff; there was also a clear association with Caius College and its founder. The college's coat of arms, derived from John Caius' own emblem, contained two entwined serpents, representing the wisdom and grace through which students might come to scholarly immortality. The flame of the candle reinforces this idea of immortality, while also suggesting the illumination of the medical world through genius.*

The academic year began on 18 October, St Luke's Day, with solemn Mass in the cathedral attended by the bishop and various civic officials.

---

*It is fitting that the golden flame, and the rest of Harvey's emblem, is still visible today just above a column in a corner of the lower loggia of the courtyard of the Bo.

This was followed a few days later by another cathedral Mass to mark the inauguration of the new rector. After the service, students huddled excitedly around the cathedral entrance. When the new rector emerged they fell upon him with violence and ripped off his multi-coloured robes in a ceremony know as *vestium laceratio*. The rector sometimes tried to appease his student attackers by distributing silver coins in all directions, but rarely to much effect.

The medical degree at Padua placed great emphasis on practical experience. Students were obliged to shadow an experienced physician for at least a year, accompanying him on his visits to the sick in Padua's San Francesco hospital. There the student learned the arts of diagnosis and prognosis, mastered the physician's bedside manner and acquired the skill of compiling case notes. The eminently pragmatic Northern European students valued this aspect of Padua's course: 'We do not lack for lecturers at home,' a councillor of the German Nation said, 'and we also have books . . . It is the study of practice that has led us to cross many mountains and at such great expense.'

Harvey threw himself with customary ardour into the hospital rounds, examining patients closely, listening to their complaints good-humouredly, and acquiring an eagle eye for recognizing ailments. He recalled treating a Paduan boy whose penis had been bitten by a dog and which had afterwards retracted, in a way 'usual in eunuchs'. To the rustic yeoman's son, his genitals seemed to resemble those of 'a monkey: two stones and no yearde'. Harvey also encountered a Venetian courtesan whose syphilitic ulcers slowly ate away at her stomach. The hospital was often packed with ailing courtesans, some of whom, one English visitor said, 'even in the midst of their tortures, are not very modest, & when they begin to be well, plainely lew'd'.

'There are', an English student remarked of San Francesco's patients, 'the most miserable & deplorable objects to exercise upon, both of men & women, young & old.' These wretched creatures underwent the tortures of 'trepanning, launcing, salivating, sweating &c' often at the hands of inexperienced students. 'I observed [terrible] things', Harvey remarked, 'with much nausea, loathing and foetor' adding that he had tried, but failed, to forget them. The noxious smells especially disturbed him, as he struggled to overcome a novice's squeamishness.

Students were also taught the art of making up medicines from plants and herbs. In the south of the city, the first physick (or botanical) garden in Europe had been laid out in 1546 at the cost of the students in physick and philosophy, 'that they might the more commodiously search into the nature & virtue of every Medicinal Herb'. Referred to as the 'garden of simples', because medicines were derived from plants in their natural or simple state, without additional concoction, the garden boasted a profusion of rare and colourful flowers and herbs, and long avenues of variegated trees.

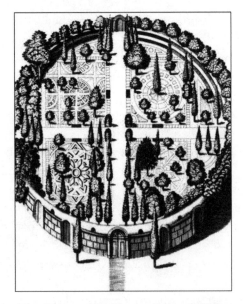

The Botanical Garden at Padua (1654).

The garden had been designed in the shape of a perfect circle enclosed by a square. The circle was divided into quadrants, with fanciful circular-shaped beds inside: a graceful and complex play of geometrical forms and flourishing nature. A conduit had been built in the garden, so that the plants were furnished with a constant supply of water from the nearby River Bacchigliano.

Other aspects of the medical degree were more familiar to the Englishman. Academic exercises took the conventional form of disputations and lectures. The pomp that accompanied formal disputations was however, remarkable, even by Cambridge standards. As a prologue, the university statutes were read out in their entirety, in Venetian dialect, the interminable litany of laws being punctuated at intervals by the rasp of a chorus of trumpets.

The Paduan syllabus was largely based on the works of Aristotle, almost half of all lectures involving the reading, and glossing, of the Greek philosopher's writings. Aristotle had always reigned supreme in the university. In 1306 Peter of Abano had been one of the first professors of medicine to teach him in the original language and one sixteenth-century English student described his Paduan tutors as 'philosophers into whom the mind of Aristotle seems to have migrated'.

Cesare Cremonini (1550–1631), chief professor of philosophy at Padua, had inherited the mantle of 'Aristotle's reincarnation' and was regarded throughout Europe as the true keeper of the flame. Harvey must have attended the compulsory lectures of the thin Italian, his bulbous head and dark, sunken eyes clearly visible to the Englishman from the front row of the low-ceilinged lecture hall at the Bo, where he sat beside the other councillors.

Cremonini's lectures were popular because they were provocative. He loved to rail against the Jesuit order, blaming them for the demise of intellectual culture in Europe. Such bombshells surprised members of the English Nation, unaccustomed to hearing controversial pronouncements from the lectern. Cremonini's style was as flamboyant as his subjects were incendiary; an author of poems and plays, and a prince of witty paradox in the dining rooms of the city, he brought students into a vivid understanding of Aristotle's ideas through his elegant epigrams and dazzling rhetorical flourishes.

Cremonini's close personal identification with the Greek philosopher also facilitated his students' understanding: he showed them
what it meant to see the world through Aristotle's eyes.

Aristotle had, Crenonini explained to the students, sought to
identify the purposes or essences of the phenomena around him.
'Men do not know a thing', he quoted the Greek, 'until they have
grasped the "why" of it (which is to grasp its final cause).' Students
of natural philosophy* should, he declared, fathom the final cause
of everyday, universal phenomena, such as a falling stone. In the
'ordinary course' of events, a stone fell because its 'nature' impelled
it towards the centre of the universe—that was its ultimate purpose.
If it was seen to swing in the air, some force must be impeding its
natural progress, and that force should be investigated. Without
understanding the 'why' of things, there could, Cremonini said, be
no knowledge of philosophical value. Anyone who merely produced
an account of the dimensions of a particular entity, for example,
covered only its 'material' cause. Such data might allow one to
speculate on the probable efficient, final or formal causes of a
phenomenon, but it offered no philosophic certainty.

In this context Cremonini often poured scorn on Padua's school
of anatomy, made famous by Vesalius some sixty years previously.
It is a sign of a weakness of the brain, he scoffed, for anatomists
to gather myriad empirical details about the internal organs that
are of no philosophic value. Anatomists, he said, boasted that

---

*Natural philosophy, or the philosophic investigation of the workings of
nature, was regarded as a theoretical rather than a practical branch of
philosophy. It aimed to furnish explanations for natural phenomena, and
to allow the student to reason about the universe in a philosophic way. It
is often described as a forerunner of modern physics or natural science but
its philosophic content renders such comparisons unhelpful. Paduan natural
philosophy might be described as the investigation of the physical world
through Aristotelian principles and methods. The first ever professor of
natural philosophy was Cremonini's predecessor at Padua, Jacopo Zabarella,
an ardent Aristotelian. It is worth bearing in mind that, throughout his life,
Harvey always identified himself as a natural philosopher.

their subject was 'the foundation of all medicine' but how could that be so when it was not grounded in the universal and rational principles of Aristotle's natural philosophy? As an instrument for the other arts the study might have its place, but it was not a serious discipline in itself: 'it is for the fool to collect trivia', Cremonini thundered, not for 'philosophical geniuses' such as himself.

As a corrective to the empirical approach of the anatomists, Cremonini offered the vision of Aristotle, who had left a significant space for particulars, and inductive enquiry, within his writings, always placing it, however, within a broader philosophic context. That space gave natural philosophers considerable scope for investigation based on observation, allowing them to infer general, philosophically valid laws from individual instances. Only by treading this particular intellectual path, he claimed, could the University of Padua fulfill its destiny and revive the 'glory of Athens'.

The English councillor in the front row of the hall could not have failed to be roused by this giddy rhetoric. He was certainly invigorated by the broader philosophical debates the lecturer outlined, and especially intrigued by Aristotle's subtle and complex opinion on the relationship between singulars and universals. It was a stance that he would one day embrace as his own.

A dissection of sacred hearts, feeling hearts, and thinking hearts

THE CATHOLIC CHURCH reverenced the heart above all other organs. The 'Sacred Heart' of Jesus, often depicted pierced by an arrow, was an object of fervent devotion in Renaissance Italy. Representations of it adorned the walls of Padua's churches, and public processions dedicated to the cult took place in the city on feast days during the year. 'Sacred Heart of Jesus,' the faithful prayed, 'we place all our trust in thee.'

Catholics believed that saints' hearts were miraculously engraved with images of Christ's Passion, such as the crucifix and the crown of thorns. When a saint died his heart was removed, embalmed and put on display, where it could be prayed to as a miracle-working relic. St Anthony, the thirteenth-century Portuguese Franciscan who became the patron saint of Padua, was closely associated with the organ. According to hagiography, Anthony attended the funeral of an avaricious usurer, during which he experienced a violent inspiration. In the middle of the service he demanded that the corpse be buried outside the city walls rather than in hallowed ground, his reason being that the usurer's body contained no heart. In accordance with Jesus' saying 'where your treasure is, there also is your heart', Anthony declared that the man's heart would be found inside his coffers rather than in his body. Friends and family left to search the man's treasure; there they discovered a heart, still warm, among the cold coins. Surgeons were sent for to perform an autopsy on the usurer's corpse; opening up his ribs they were unable to find his heart.

This extraordinary scene is depicted in a famous rectangular bronze relief inside Padua's five-domed Basilica of St Anthony, which rises up out of the teeming alleyways and markets of the middle islet of the city. The relief, wrought by Donatello in the fifteenth century, adorns the basilica's high altar.

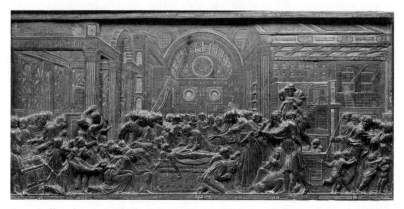

Donatello's bronze relief of the *Miracle of the man with the avaricious heart.*

Donatello offers an intensely dramatic vignette featuring an extensive cast of characters. The main protagonists are St Anthony, around whom members of the crowd prostrate themselves in prayer, and the anatomist, frozen in the act of opening up the thorax of the usurer with his knife. Some of the onlookers crowd around the surgeon, peering down eagerly at the corpse; others recoil in horror. The perspective, and the movement and momentum of the crowd, draw our attention to the very centre of the image, its heartless heart, as it were—the open and empty body prostrate beneath the anatomist's hand. Donatello is said to have drawn inspiration from anatomies he attended at Padua University; if that is true then he was one of the first of many Renaissance artists to study anatomy in a bid to produce representations of the body which were more detailed than those of their medieval predecessors.

There are several other altars in the basilica, one of which houses relics of Anthony's body. During Harvey's time in Padua, a perpetual line of pilgrims would queue up to pray to these relics, which were believed to have the power of curing physical diseases (some of them associated with the heart), and of expelling evil spirits that had conquered the hearts of 'demoniacal persons'. In the hushed Gothic gloom of the church's candlelit interior, the possessed prostrated themselves close by Anthony's relics in the hope of a release from their torments, a priest standing over them, muttering the prayers of exorcism, his hands joined together against his heart.

According to popular Catholic belief, during his life a man wrote on his heart, the organ being as it were a book where all his deeds were recorded. After his death, man ascended to the House of Judgement, where God would open up and read his heart. Having examined the volume the eternal judge would pronounce sentence on the man—a certain length of time in purgatory, or permanent residence in heaven or hell—as though appending a moral at the end of a book. The heart was thus both the symbol and the embodiment of man's soul.

This idea is illustrated in Padua's Scrovegni Chapel, situated to the north of the city, a single chamber twenty metres long, nine metres wide and nineteen metres high. In the fourteenth century, Giotto, the Tuscan painter who had formerly been a shepherd, decorated it with intensely dramatic frescoes celebrating the lives of Jesus and of the parents of the Virgin Mary. He dyed its vault in the deep blue of the dawn sky and studded it with golden stars. Giotto's personifications of the virtues and vices stare at one another across the nave. Envy is a blind woman with a serpent for a tongue. Among her head garments she hides her sin-stained heart, emblem of her soul, from the searching eyes of God. Opposite her the beautiful woman Charity hands her pure heart up to God, who accepts the gift readily.

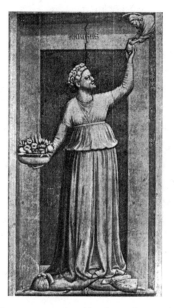

Giotto's *Charity*. Her gesture is echoed in the representation of the Last Judgement, painted on the chapel's west wall, where the figure of Enrico Scrovegni, who commissioned the building, can be seen presenting his heart to the Madonna.

Harvey was aware of the cult of the Sacred Heart, referring to an important aspect of it in his later lectures, when he discussed the wound in the side of the crucified Christ from which both blood and water had miraculously issued. He also absorbed the intense reverence for the heart so pervasive in the religious culture of the period, as he celebrated the organ in his writings as the 'tutelary deity of the body'. The religious inflection here is utterly character-istic. Contemplating the blood that moved in and out of the heart, Harvey marvelled at 'how sensitive it is to harm done to it by things that are hurtful, and to the comfort of things that cherish it'; this, he concluded, was because the liquid was the 'primary' and 'principal' residence of man's immortal soul. Harvey may have been influenced by the Aristotelian notion that the rational or spiritual soul dwelt within the heart, but he is also likely to have been drawing on the Christian tradition.

The idea that the heart was God's citadel, and the residence of man's soul, was by no means exclusive to Catholics. A preacher of the seventeenth-century Church of England declared that 'there is no veine in mee, that is not full of the blood of God's Son'; while an English religious poet of the period implored God to 'batter' his heart, in order to 'break' into his life. The heart was also reverenced as a sacred organ by radical English Protestants such as John Bunyan. In an early episode in *The Pilgrim's Progress*, the most famous Protestant allegory of the seventeenth century, the protagonist, Christian, finds himself in a parlour filled with dust. A man enters the chamber with a broom and vainly attempts to clean it. Some time later a 'damsel' arrives with some water, with which she successfully cleanses the room. The Interpreter, who stands beside Christian throughout, elucidates the symbolism of the scene: 'the parlour is the heart of the man, that has never been sanctified by the sweet grace' of God; the dust 'original sin'. The man who 'first swept is [human] law; she that brought water and did sprinkle it is the gospel'.

In the words of the Renaissance Italian prayer, the Sacred Heart of Jesus 'feels all, knows all, and thinks of all'. The notion that man felt with his heart was commonplace in the seventeenth century. The organ was regarded, in Harvey's phrase, as 'the seat and organ of all passions'—the stage where the emotional action of man's life unfolded.

Traditional Galenic physiology confirmed and encouraged this popular belief. A super-sensitive organ, the heart was said to be activated by the emotions and thereby transformed into a furnace which heated the blood. The hearts of men excited by powerful feelings would beat quickly and become instantly and intensely hot. In some cases, such as that of the Earl of Gloucester in *King Lear*, 'extremes of passion, joy and grief' might even 'burst' the heart, an exploded heart often being given as the cause of death by physicians who carried out autopsies. In contrast, the fire that burned inside the hearts of lovers produced beneficial effects: it gently heated the entire body, invigorating men and inspiring them to bold acts, and rendering even the most shrewish women warm, tender and impulsive.

If the heart moved to the rhythm of man's feelings, then it could also make the emotions dance to its music. Certain movements of the heart were believed to stir up particular humours: a vigorous beating of the organ producing choler, gentler motions, melancholy. The way a man's heart beat thus influenced his character. Naturally vigorous hearts produced irascible, choleric people, while those who possessed hearts effective in cooling the blood down were invariably slow to anger or panic, and thus generally closer to the phlegmatic or melancholic personality type.

Physiological ideas permeated everyday language. In evoking a man's character people invariably referred to his heart, describing him as 'frozen' or 'empty' hearted, and as having either a 'loving' or a 'poor' heart. Men could either be 'iron-hearted', 'lion-hearted', or 'generous of heart'. When King Lear is appalled and bemused by the cruel behaviour of his daughter Regan, he asks his surgeons to 'anatomize' her so that he can 'see what breeds about her heart'. Only then will he understand the essence of her sadistic character, as well as the cause.

While the idea of a feeling heart no longer makes physiological sense, it nevertheless survives in everyday language and so remains familiar to us. We continue to speak of 'tender' and 'stony' hearted people; we can still 'take' heart, or 'lose' heart at a sudden turn of events, and hearts will be melted, wounded and broken as long as the English language endures. The notion, however, that the Sacred Heart of Jesus could, in the words of the Italian prayer, '*know* all, and *think* of all' is utterly alien to our culture.

Yet in the seventeenth century people believed that the heart was capable of thought. The King James Bible (published in 1611) reveals that it was seen as the thinking organ par excellence, the 'mind' being named much less frequently in that regard. In the Old Testament, God gives Solomon 'a wise and understanding heart', while Job returns the compliment by praising God as 'wise in heart'. The Gospel of Luke describes the heart as the home of the 'imagination'; in Matthew man can even commit adultery in his heart. For the evangelist John, too, it is in the heart that men 'understand' and where they can be corrupted. When the Devil wants Judas to betray Jesus he puts the evil idea into the apostle's heart rather than into his head.* These New Testament references may have been partly inspired by Roman culture, in which the act of memorizing was described as 'learning by heart', and in which literature was believed to express the 'thoughts of the heart'. It was in this context that a contemporary poet described someone as having a 'naked thinking heart', and that Edmund Spenser could evoke the distress of one of the heroines of his *The Faerie Queene* by writing that 'her faint heart was with the frozen cold / Benumb'd so inly, that he wits nigh fail'd'.

In Harvey's time, the heart occupied an exalted place in the hierarchy of the organs because of its spiritual, emotional, and intellectual significance, as well as its physiological importance. When we later try to understand why a natural philosopher or anatomist might select the heart as the subject for his investigations, we must bear in mind the organ's cultural prestige. For this was a culture in which men believed, in the words of one preacher: 'How little of a Man is the *Heart* and yet [it] is all by which he *is*.'

---

* These beliefs continue to inform Catholic liturgy. During the confessional prayer, at the moment when a member of the congregation confesses that he has sinned 'in his thoughts' as well as in his words and actions, he beats his breast as though pounding his sinful heart.

5. Paduan studies II (c.1600–1602): 'The exposition of anatomy'

IN THE COLD antechamber on the first floor of the Bo, Harvey waited to be called into the circular anatomical theatre. The very first permanent theatre of its kind in Europe, it had been built in 1594, 'for the majesty of Venice', in order to 'display the glory of her nature no less than did the circus games and gymnasiums of antiquity'.* Anatomies were made free of charge, according to university statutes, 'in order that everyone may come' to enjoy what were civic as well as scholarly spectacles.

As Harvey waited, the porters called into the theatre men and women from the general public—typically a miscellaneous sample of 'teachers, tailors, shoemakers, sandal-makers, butchers, salted fish dealers, porters, basket-bearers . . . jacks-in-office, money-lenders and barbers', dressed in the colourful uniforms of their trade. The porter ushered them up the theatre's external spiral staircase, which led to a series of landings, and so out onto the upper gallery. This was the fifth of the circular galleries, in this theatre shaped like a wooden 'o'.

The public filed out into the gallery until no one else could be

* The building has indeed proved to be 'permanent', being the only theatre of the Renaissance to have survived intact to this day. The magnificent structure can still be visited at the University of Padua.

squeezed in. They peered down at the dissection table, which dominated an oval floor space of only twenty by twenty feet. The table was encircled by a halo of light emanating from two candelabra which stood at either end and eight torches held by standing students.

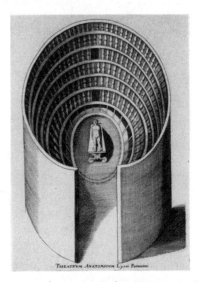

The anatomy theatre at Padua University (1654).

Each member of the 250-strong audience was wedged into a twenty-inch space in which they could stand with a tolerable degree of discomfort. Each of the five galleries was raised a full three feet above the one beneath it, the steep sides of the theatre giving it the appearance of a funnel. The press of so many people packed tightly into such a small, illuminated, windowless space, and the height of the middle and upper galleries, induced in some spectators nausea and vertigo. Carved wooden railings prevented queasy members of the audience falling forwards, down on to the dissection table. It was impossible, however, for anyone suddenly taken ill to leave the theatre without the entire row filing out before them. For the duration of the three-hour dissection, the spectator was hemmed in.

The porters called in the gowned medical students next, nation by nation, the Germans being particularly well represented. They climbed the external stairs and took their places in the fourth, third and second galleries, below the public. When they had finally settled, it was Harvey's turn to enter, along with the other councillors, who had the privilege of occupying the first gallery.

Anatomical demonstrations required a cold venue so that the cadaver did not putrefy too quickly. They were usually held in January or February, at Carnival time (ironically the word 'carnival' comes from the Latin *carnelevamen*, which means to 'put away flesh'). Sessions began in the bitter chill of the Paduan winter morning, not long after the ringing of the eight o'clock bells; this particular anatomy would have taken place in February 1601 or 1602.

After a few minutes the porters called for silence and announced the entrance of the rectors of the city and of the university, attired in their robes of purple and gold. They were followed by local aristocrats, government officials and university professors, all of whom were likewise dressed in magnificent robes. They took their seats immediately around the dissection table and in the *luoghi a basso*—small boxes directly beneath the first gallery. If any waggish student had trespassed into these areas before the arrival of the dignitaries, he was ejected and fined. It was vital that, at this important civic occasion, people sat 'according to the degrees of their precedence'.

It was the duty of the porters to ensure that the proper calm and modesty reigned throughout the auditorium; they hovered on the landings, ever ready to quell trouble. They were specifically instructed, in the statutes, to 'restrain the importunate plebs', who were forbidden to chat or laugh while the anatomist spoke. On no account should there be any sudden movement or speaking out. In particular, 'during the demonstrations of the female genitalia, they should contemplate everything with chaste eyes'. Yet despite their best efforts, heckling often occurred; on occasion, spectators even fell to blows.

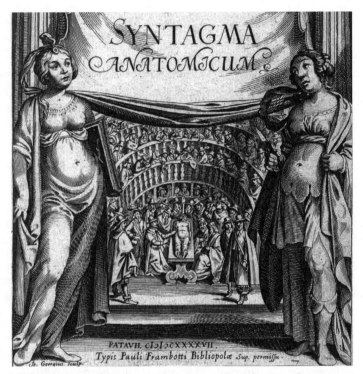

Engraving of the anatomy theatre at Padua on the title page of an anatomical volume (1647). The public in the upper galleries resembles the audience of a play. Men and women loll around, and appear to talk to one another.

A far greater threat of disturbance came, however, from the students. During anatomies they sometimes fought duels with swords. There were also loud slanging matches between the various nations, with the 'mad Italians' (as they were known) regularly taunting the others. Objects, as well as insults, were hurled across the auditorium; on one occasion a melon struck a professor full in the face. The anatomist often became 'confused, upset and bewildered owing to some noise and disorder that the students made'; he would then hurry quickly to the end of a dissection, or walk out before the conclusion. Offending students were fined heavily for causing trouble, and stripped of their voting privileges.

The theatre had been designed with the express aim of limiting disturbances, its magnificent structure and atmosphere enveloping the civic and religious ritual of anatomy in an air of solemnity. Its walls were adorned with the imposing emblems of the Venetian Republic as well as the various insignia of the illustrious anatomists who performed there. The limited space inside the galleries made it difficult for spectators to turn to their neighbours; the darkness precluded the identification of other audience members.

The auditorium was also filled with the sweet airs of music, played on lutes to quell the 'tumult and stomping' of the spectators and 'to raise them from their sad look'. The melodies were similar to those played on other civic occasions requiring an atmosphere of tranquillity.

The lute players were among the last to enter the theatre, taking their seats around the dissection table. Now that all the spectators were present, the head porter, carrying a golden mace, entered the auditorium and demanded silence. He announced the arrival of the protagonist of the performance, using his Latinized name 'Hieronymous Fabricius ab Aquapendente'. Fabricius (born Girolamo Fabrizi) was professor of anatomy and surgery at Padua. Dressed in dazzling purple and gold robes, he entered with a theatrical flourish to the accompaniment of music, followed by two assistants. Still brimming with energy in his late sixties, the anatomist marched over towards the throne of carved wood next to the dissection table, then slowly lowered himself into it. His two assistants took their places on stools beside him.

Fabricius' robes were identical to those of the rector, a unique privilege among the University faculty past and present, granted him by Venice. The small, bald-headed, bearded anatomist wore these garments with the ease of one who had been born a noble, then risen to the very top of his profession. Fabricius was renowned throughout Europe as the latest in a line of great Paduan anatomists which included Andreas Vesalius and Gabriele Fallopius, discoverer of the Fallopian tubes. Along with the robes, the 'most serene' republic awarded Fabricius a substantial salary, as well as a golden chain. Venice also constructed the new permanent anatomical theatre at his behest, and perhaps also to his specifications.*

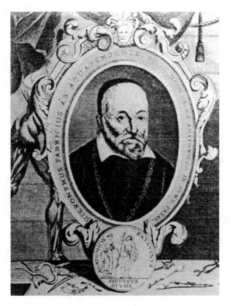

Seventeenth-century portrait of Fabricius.

Members of the German Nation, however, were less than impressed with their professor, complaining that the *caro vecchione* ('dear old man') had become arrogant, vain and indolent in his dotage, 'like a lazy horse who had to be spurred on'. Fabricius responded to their proddings by finding every possible excuse to delay or even cancel his public dissections, at the shortest possible

---

*Famous for his genius in anatomy, Fabricius was also notorious for his choleric disposition. One day a former student of his, newly promoted within the faculty to the same professorial rank as Fabricius, refused to give way to his old mentor on the city's pavements. Fabricius responded by hiring armed bodyguards to escort him everywhere. Should he be insulted by the upstart a second time, he would demonstrate that 'he could handle a knife in other ways than in dissecting cadavers'.

notice. When, at a meeting of the university authorities, the Germans protested about his behaviour, the anatomist claimed not to understand them on account of their appalling Latin pronunciation. 'It's a great shame', he sneered, 'that you Germans compress your lips so much while speaking, so that the fs come out as vs; one hardly understands you.' Fabricius then proceeded to impersonate them, much to the amusement of everyone present.

According to the university statutes, the anatomical performance should be conducted along traditional lines, with the seated professor reading from Mondino, the *sector* doing the cutting, and the *ostensor* indicating to the audience the organs the professor described. Yet Fabricius insisted that very little cutting be carried out in the theatre, always instructing his assistants to dissect the body before the performance. They worked upon the corpse in a little white stone chamber, situated directly beneath the auditorium, where all the skeletons, instruments, sponges and clothes were stored.

The illustrious anatomist now called for the cadaver. To the accompaniment of lutes, the body was handed up to his assistants from the dissection pit through a trapdoor. The assistants positioned it carefully on the brown seven-foot dissection table, where it lay at the very centre of the circular theatre.

Fabricius now addressed the audience. 'The exposition of anatomy is sacred and divine, it must be approached in the same spirit and mind as divine service, since it bears witness to the power, goodness and wisdom of God. For God wishes and has the power to ensure that all parts of the human body and those of every animal are in the best possible situation, and that all parts of man are in the very best state. Such marvels of nature should not lie hidden from us, so we shall now reveal them.'

The aim of natural philosophy was to understand God, and to uncover his laws, through an investigation of His created world. Fabricius was concerned to show that anatomy could play a crucial part in this noblest of all endeavours. Perhaps partly provoked by

Cremonini's dismissal of the subject as an empirical enterprise of little deductive value, he aimed to raise anatomy's philosophical prestige, and his own profile in the process, by demonstrating how it could be conducted along Aristotelian lines and to Aristotelian ends. The magnificent theatre that had been built for him embodied these ambitions.

'I shall follow and expound Aristotle,' Fabricius announced, 'that great interpreter of nature.' A representative man of the Renaissance, the Italian wanted to revive an intellectual project of the classical world in its original, uncorrupted form. Drawing on the plethora of freshly edited Aristotelian texts spawned by the printing press, he would dissect *as if he were* Aristotle—that is, as though Galen had not yet been born.

Aristotle had viewed the body as the 'soul-in-action', which was to say that the soul used a particular organ as its instrument for a specific end. The Aristotelian anatomist must identify the various 'causes' of an organ if he was to define what 'kind-of-a-thing' it was. The first step was to provide a description or *historia* of an organ. Next, its action (or 'efficient cause') was to be understood (this included an investigation of the particular role it performed within the body's economy). Then the structure (or 'material cause') of the organ was to be considered, for this enabled the organ to perform its action. Lastly, the 'final cause' or purpose of the organ was to be identified. Following Aristotle, and in contrast to Galen, Fabricius examined an organ (or groups of organs) in isolation from each other, dedicating a single anatomy session to, say, the organs of sight, sound, speech, reproduction or respiration.

On this occasion we may imagine Fabricius investigating the eye, his assistant removing one from the cadaver's head. As it was held up to the audience, the anatomist offered a detailed description, drawing on anatomical authorities and his own observations, before explaining its function within the body. Turning to its structure and substance—its crystalline humour, for example—he showed how it was designed in order to fulfil its function. Finally he declared that the purpose of the organ, its *raison d'être*, was seeing. This final cause allowed one to fully grasp its form and action, for it had been designed by God with that express purpose in mind.

At this point, Fabricius called for the body of an animal to be passed up from the dissection pit. His Aristotelian aim was to investigate the function and purpose of an organ in *all* animals, or rather to define *the* universal organ in *the* animal that was man, plus every other animal—man being an animal in physical or material terms. Fabricius, following his Greek master, held that only in this way could the anatomist arrive at generalized philosophical knowledge of an organ—the detailed investigations of a variety of different animals leading to universalized knowledge. It was through this subtle interplay between particulars and general statements (as well as through his use of the four causes) that Fabricius aimed to give the lie to Cremonini's criticisms of anatomy.

Fabricius' assistants hauled up, out of the trap door, the carcass of a sheep, then removed one of its eyes. Fabricius described it, comparing it to the human organ already examined. He then asked his assistants to bring up further animal carcasses—of a bird, oxen or bull—from the dissection pit. Examining the eye of each in turn, Fabricius described their differences and similarities, in order to build up a generalized picture of how all animals see. Having finished with a particular animal specimen, its remains were thrown into a large bucket that lay beside the dissection table.

The highpoints of Fabricius' anatomical spectacles from the public's point of view, were the presentation of the naked, partially opened corpse at the beginning, and the ripping up of the menagerie. The sight of the dead animals probably struck them as absurd and amusing, as though a civic theatre had been transformed into a butcher's shop. Intermittent ripples of excitement went through the upper galleries at these strange sights; people gasped, and chatted away. The professors and dignitaries at the front of the theatre may also have regarded the exploration of animal carcasses as incongruous, as it was not common practice in conventional university anatomy.

Yet as the three-hour demonstration progressed, the public became increasingly insensitive to shock, as well as to the lulling effects of the music. The sound of their murmuring gradually rose; they fidgeted in their confined places. To muffle their noise, the musicians would be asked to increase the volume. In some universities a fool was also employed to raise the audience's flagging spirits. A wooden panel in one of the galleries suddenly opened, revealing the fool's funny face. He cracked an outrageous joke, perhaps about the corpse, then quickly popped his head back inside the panel, shutting the door with a slam.

In the middle galleries many of the students also become restive, but from irritation rather than boredom. For one thing, they could hardly see the body parts Fabricius was discussing, only the vaguest outline being visible from the third and fourth galleries. More importantly, virtually all of them had enrolled at Padua with an eye to a career as a surgeon or physician. What they had hoped for was a crash course in practical dissection and surgical techniques, and a thorough description of the human body, within the context of physiology and medicine. Vesalius, who worked within the human-centred, Galenic anatomical tradition, had secured Padua's fame sixty years previously with this variety of instruction.

'I lament the fate of myself and my fellow students', the councillor of the German Nation moaned to the university authorities, 'and marvel at the good luck of my predecessors. They often saw two or three bodies dissected [completely] each year, while we who have come here at no less expense cannot even see one. Fabricius has already spent two months describing the bones of the head. Now that he has reached the muscles, he has devoted three hours to three of them, and there are so many muscles that two years will not be sufficient. When will he talk about the viscera?' The 'dear old man', with his irrelevant philosophical ideas and his esoteric comparisons between human and animal organs, was simply too slow. He also progressed, or rather digressed, in 'a confused and disorderly way [discussing] a detached arm one day, many days later the foot. I don't see how anyone can learn the relations of the parts to the whole'.

Predictably, the complaints only roused Fabricius' sarcasm. 'This Fabricius', the imperious anatomist whined, mimicking the Germans' inelegant Latin, 'can teach nothing usefully, nothing productively', emphasizing the vulgarity of the words 'useful' and 'productive' to a natural philosopher intent on understanding God's creation. The Germans, he declared, were utterly unworthy of his masterful performances. Henceforth he delayed or cancelled the sessions evermore frequently and flagrantly, so that the German students were forced to hire rival anatomists to conduct private anatomies, in the Galenic–Vesalian style, in makeshift outdoor theatres around the city.

Yet what the Germans deemed arcane and irrelevant was music to the ears of the alert, diminutive Englishman who would sit in the first gallery of the theatre, in the penumbra of the ring of candlelight surrounding the dissection table, listening to the master's every word, committing to memory his methods and ideas. Harvey must have sensed that he was in the presence of a man who, through his Aristotelian principles and comparative approach, had 'placed his head among the stars' of the intellectual firmament.

The cadaver used at public anatomies would, preferably, be whole, and of a young and healthy person, with a well-defined and well-maintained musculature. Ideally, it would be the corpse of a criminal hanged in Padua; if none was available then anyone executed in the Venetian Republic or in Italy would suffice. The criminals could not themselves hail from the Veneto, for the dissection of their corpses might give offence to their relatives and potentially lead to a vociferous protest in the theatre; nor could the cadaver be of noble birth. In some Italian cities, it was preferred to perform dissections on the bodies of 'Jews or other infidels'.

Dissection constituted part of the punishment for 'delinquents' who had exiled themselves from human society and sympathy by their felonies. Closely resembling the quartering of a body after hanging, anatomy added a new terror to death, especially for those who believed in the resurrection of the body in some form, as all Catholics did. At the beginning of his anatomy Fabricius would solemnly announce 'our subject for the anatomy lesson has been hanged', indicating that the dissection was an epilogue to the execution.

Prior to the hanging of a felon earmarked for dissection, a messenger from the university would visit the monks who attended him during his final hours. The messenger carried with him a mandate from the rector and the city governor, demanding that the body be given up to the university immediately following the execution. The order was kept secret from the criminal, so as not to provoke hysteria or any blasphemous utterances on the gallows. After the execution the body might be carried to the university on a bier in procession by the monks, or collected directly from the scaffold by a group of students. Sometimes students tied the corpse to a horse's tail and dragged it all the way to the Bo.

The close cooperation between the religious orders, the state and the university demanded by these operations, sometimes bordered on collusion. During one dissection of the period, the anatomist announced 'tomorrow we shall have another body—I believe they will [today] hang a man upon which I shall demonstrate to you'—which suggests that executions were possibly timed with anatomies in mind. Anatomical needs probably influenced the type of execution decreed by a judge (a hanged criminal was the most suitable for an anatomy) and may even have affected the sentence itself. In Bologna it was rumoured that one 'poor wretch had been condemned to prison for life, but to satisfy the demands of the scholars, the cardinal legate overruled the sentence and had him condemned to death'.

When cadavers were unavailable through official channels, students would steal them from hospitals and graveyards, bringing them stealthily to the Bo by night, often with the approval, and participation, of their professors. Sometimes cadavers were even filched during funerals, the students whisking them off biers, or out of open graves, and sprinting away to the university with their prize. On one occasion, hearing word of the murder of a peasant, students 'hurried to the scene to obtain the cadaver for an anatomy; but the peasants having gathered there in good number did not let them take the body away, and the scholars were obliged to be patient'.

After a demonstration had finished, the cadaver (if no longer of use for a future dissection) was consigned to a religious institution. If monks had originally delivered the body to the university, they would now come to collect it. With the help of the students, they conveyed it to their monastery, where it would receive a Christian burial. As the executed person had been subjected to the appalling ignominy of dissection, more than twenty Masses would be celebrated for their soul. That, at least, was how the cadaver was supposed to be disposed of according to the law. In Padua, however, the students were notorious for hurling the remains of dissected cadavers into the river, or feeding them to the dogs, along with the carcasses of the animals Fabricius had cut up.

On 25 April 1602 Harvey presented himself for the final oral examination of his medical degree in the presence of a Palatine count. Venice had bestowed on the count the power of conferring degrees, even on non-Catholics such as Harvey, much to the annoyance of the Vatican.

'Count Sigismund', according to Harvey's diploma, 'listened with pleasure to the noble and erudite William Harvey of Folkestone, an Englishman, son of the illustrious Thomas Harvey, Councillor of the English Nation, learnedly, eloquently, and in a praiseworthy and excellent style, discussing the themes in Arts and Medicine propounded him by . . . Hieronymus Fabricius ab Aquapendente, Public Professor of Anatomy and Surgery [and various other professors] . . . moreover subtly replying to, and lucidly resolving the argument, doubts, and cases brought before him.'

The examination took the form of a disputation, the eager Englishman defending his theories in front of Fabricius and company, with agile arguments demonstrating both his grasp of philosophical logic and his mastery of rhetorical style. After the interrogation one of the professors 'did solemnly decorate and adorn the noble William Harvey with the accustomed Insignia and ornaments belonging to a Doctor'. A golden ring was placed on his finger, and the cap of a doctor on his head as a 'sign of the Crown of Virtue'. Then Harvey was presented with 'certain books of philosophy and medicine', the professor opening and closing them in front of his eyes before 'bestowing on him the Kiss of Peace with the Magistral Benediction'. This intriguing ceremonial gesture probably symbolized Harvey's mastery of natural philosophy and medicine, disciplines that were now 'open books' to him.

By this ceremony the Paduan authorities placed their official seal on Harvey's 'authority and liberty . . . in every country and place to lecture, repeat, advise, heal, debate, interpret, to decide questions, to govern schools [and] make bachelors'. He had won the right to teach and practise as a physician, and to embark on a potentially lucrative career.

Thomas Harvey also basked in his eldest son's brilliance, being described in the diploma as 'illustrious' rather than as a simple 'yeoman'. Whatever moral degradations the stern patriarch may have feared for William on his departure to Italy, he must have been well pleased to greet the young man who returned, diploma and books in hand, to 'Kent and Christendom' in 1602.

6. Early years in London (c.1602– c.1610): 'Begin the world'

A FTER PASSING SEVERAL months with his family in the quiet of Kent, Harvey journeyed north to London. A bustling city of 150,000 souls, London boasted ten times more inhabitants than any other city in England, and would soon become the largest capital in Europe. Harvey settled in the very heart of the maze-like medieval city, near to Ludgate, a stone's throw from both St Paul's and the Thames at Blackfriars' Stairs.

Some time after Harvey's arrival, James I, recently crowned king of England after Elizabeth's death in 1603, pressed him for a forced loan, as was the prerogative of the Crown. Harvey was able to avoid the imposition by claiming lack of funds. 'Whereas it hath pleased His Majesty', his official supplication reads, 'to direct his privy seal to William Harvey doctor of physic for to borrow of him six pounds and thirteen shillings and fourpence, we certify that the said Doctor Harvey is a young man whose father is yet living [i.e. he had to be provided for] and that being to begin the world his means and abilities are such as he is unfit to lend'.

Harvey presented himself as a young adventurer, who had only just set forth on the journey of his life. One of his first steps was to get himself a well-off and well-connected wife. His marriage licence is dated 24 November 1604. 'William Harvie a batcheler aged xxvi yeres or there abowts of the parishe of St Martins by Ludgate allegeth that he intendeth to maray one Elizabeth Browne mayden aged xxiiii the naturall and lawfull daughter of Lancelot Browne Doctor of Phisicke [who] appeared personally before the Judge [and] giveth his expresse consent hereunto. And then appeared Thomas Harvye of the Towne of Folston [Folkestone] naturall father unto the said William Harvie and giveth his consent.'

Harvey's alliance with the Browne family created a number of opportunities. His father-in-law, Lancelot Browne, was a fellow of both St John's College, Cambridge and the College of Physicians in London. He was also connected at court, being physician to King James. Browne evidently believed that the prosperous Kentish yeoman family could keep his daughter in a manner which became her status, Thomas Harvey's gift to the newlyweds of the manor of Boxtall Lane, Kent, doubtless inspiring confidence. He also saw professional promise in his sharp ambitious son-in-law. Within months of the marriage, Browne was promoting William's cause at court, recommending him for the post of physician to the Tower of London. In a letter to the influential Earl of Salisbury, he vouched for his son-in-law's 'good learninge', 'loyallty', 'discretion' and 'honesty'. 'Yf any doubtfull matter of moment in physik should occur in his practice there', he also assured the earl, 'he should have me always readie to resolve him therein.'

Many years later, in one of his published writings, Harvey painted a vignette of his wife Elizabeth which breathes affection, humour and sensuality:

> My wife had an excellent, and well instructed Parrat [i.e. parrot], which was long her delight . . . he was permitted to walk at liberty through the whole house . . . If she called him, he would make answer, and flying to her, would grasp her garments with his claws, and bill . . . [I] alwaies thought him to be a Cock-parrat, by his notable excellence in singing and talking. For amongst birds . . . [only] the males charm the females by the pleasant musick of their voice, and allure them to pay their homage to Venus . . . Many times when he was sportive and wanton, he would sit in her lap.

In matters of reproduction, Harvey believed that, 'Nature tends to perfection'. Consequently, in choosing a bed partner, 'we ought', he advised friends, 'to consult more with our sense and instinct, than our reason, and prudence, and Interest . . . a blessing goes with a marriage for love upon a strong impulse'. Yet William and Elizabeth's marriage was not blessed with children and childlessness carried with it an acute social stigma. It was the duty of 'honest' men to marry, have children, and become the providers for, and masters of, their households. They must also produce grandchildren for their fathers and so extend the family line. Childbearing was the *raison d'être* of women, who were more or less confined to the home.

Lancelot Browne doubtless assisted his son-in-law with his application to become a member of the College of Physicians, an institution where patronage went a long way. The college had been established in the reign of Henry VIII to oversee the practice of medicine within, and just outside, the city. Thomas Linacre was its founder and first president; John Caius had also served in that office. The college, which comprised a small elite of around forty fellows, enjoyed a monopoly over medicine in London, having the exclusive right to grant licences to physicians, as well as to legally prosecute unlicensed empirics or quack practitioners—amateurs whose treatments were based on experience rather than learning.

Distinguished on the one hand from surgeons and barbers, who treated the exterior of the body, and on the other from apothecaries, who made up drugs, physicians diagnosed patients and prescribed internal medicines, such as pills, foods and enemas. Customarily, surgeons and apothecaries were obliged to follow a physician's instructions, rather than diagnose or treat a patient independently.

Physicians enjoyed a far more exalted status than their colleagues. This was reflected in the long purple gowns they were permitted to wear; in parish registers where they were respectfully referred to as 'Masters'; and in the extortionate fees they could charge. As much as £75 could be demanded for a 'guaranteed cure', at a time when the wage of a maidservant was around £3 a year. In a city ravaged periodically by smallpox, tuberculosis and the plague, physicians were in short supply and great demand, and there were plenty of desperate patients willing to pay their vast fees.

On 4 May 1603 Harvey left his Ludgate home, walked south down Crede Lane (named after the writers and publishers of religious works who dwelt there) then turned east into busy Carter Lane, passing its large-fronted houses. Next he descended Do-little Lane, so called because of the absence of shops there, before turning right into Knyght Ryder Street at the sign of the Boar's Head tavern, famed for the medieval knights who had congregated there before moving off to their jousts in Smithfield.

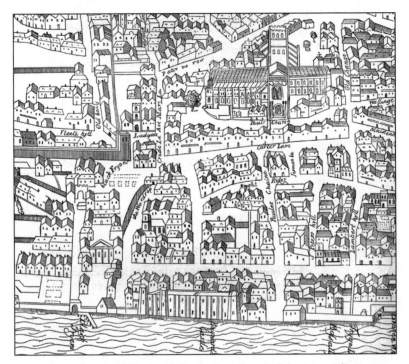

Map of London (c.1570) formerly attributed to Ralph Agas. This section shows the journey from Harvey's home to Knyght Ryder Street.

As Harvey paced through the narrow lanes, he was surrounded by the eternal uproar of the unresting city. Street cries confronted him on every corner 'Old shoes for new brooms'; 'Ripe cherries, ripe!' Tradesmen had to shout to be heard above the tumult of 'hammers beating in one place, tubs hooping in another, pots clanking in a third'. The country boy must have been struck by the intense press of people in the streets: 'men, women and children meet in such shoals', one observer recorded, 'that posts are set up of purpose to strengthen the houses, lest with jostling one another they should shoulder them down'. He would also have remarked on the eclectic character of the Londoners: 'Foot by foot and elbow by elbow' walked 'the knight, the gallant, the upstart, the gentleman, the clown, the pimp, the beggar, the scholar, the puritan, the thief, the blackamoor, the Italian, the country bumpkin.'

In Knyght Ryder Street, Harvey identified the headquarters of the College of Physicians, a tiny stone house only twenty-four feet high and wide, bequeathed to the institution by Thomas Linacre. Entering the building he was ushered into a small room where four or five seated censors (or examiners) and the president of the college awaited him. They were dressed in purple robes and silk purple caps; those who found the spring day cool wore their velvet cloaks also.

Harvey presented himself with a bow as a doctor of medicine in the University of Padua, no doubt brandishing his impressive diploma. The college accepted only university-trained men who had mastered traditional medical theory and whose Latin was sound. 'You will be examined', the president informed him, 'and make answer in Latin'. (At this point certain candidates, who had trained as apprentice surgeons or apothecaries rather than at university, claimed that they had forgotten their Latin as a result of illness). 'What is an element?' the first censor began. 'How many temperaments are there?' enquired the second. The questions then came at Harvey relentlessly, 'What is epilepsy?'

'What is colic?' 'What are the causes of ague?'

'Anyone wishing to be admitted', Harvey was told, 'must be well read in Galen. Are you familiar with the editions of Caius and Linacre?' To satisfy the censors on this point, Harvey was asked: 'Pray, read to me a little from this Latin Galen.' The college, Harvey learned, regarded Galen's writings as the equivalent of Holy Writ. Any candidate championing alternative approaches to medical treatment was viewed with extreme suspicion, those not sufficiently *au fait* with the writings of the master were turned away with the instruction to study him with greater diligence. When the examination was over, the censors declared Harvey's 'replies to all questions' 'entirely satisfactory'. 'Nevertheless', he was informed, 'your suit will be put off until another time, with our tacit admission to practise.'

Harvey underwent three further examinations. He 'did answere so readily and fully withall' on these occasions that 'the whole company did both admire him, and took very singular lyking unto him'. In October 1604, he achieved admittance as a *licentiatus*, an intermediate stage before full fellowship, which carried with it official permission to practise. Harvey paid £11 3s 4d for the privilege, along with a subscription of £4 for his first year.

On 16 May 1607, Harvey was summoned once again to the hall in Knyght Ryder Street. When he arrived he found the president of the college and fourteen other fellows waiting for him. Harvey stood before them as the college statutes were recited, along with its table of fines. 'Any fellows revealing college secrets will be compelled to pay 10s; those found consulting with an unlicensed apothecary will be fined the same'; fellows must never speak disrespectfully of Galen. Harvey took a solemn oath to adhere to these decrees, as the fellows dressed him in the purple robe of the fully-fledged fellow. Harvey then shook each fellow by the hand before taking his place, for the first time, among them.

Some college business was transacted before the fellows retired to another room where they feasted on sweetmeats and wine. Harvey had to settle the reckoning for the banquet, which cost £5 11s 8d. It was a sizeable bill, but he and his father would have realized that such expenses were shrewd investments. As part of a rising professional elite, he would soon be a gentleman, in wealth if not in name.

Harvey rose effortlessly through the college ranks, being appointed censor (an office reserved, according to the statutes, for 'the best, wisest, and most descreet' among the fellowship) then treasurer. Ultimately he became one of the college 'Elects' who had the power to choose the president. A loyal and energetic member of the body, Harvey persecuted quacks with customary ardour and efficiency, severely reprimanding those who criticized either the college or medical authorities such as Galen.

Harvey also used to the full the power vested in him to 'search, survey, and prove whether medicines, wares [of] drugs, in shops belonging to the art and mystery of the apothecary be wholesome meet and fit for the cure, health, and ease of His Majesty's subjects'. He and his colleagues would raid up to thirty apothe-cary's shops in a single day. Walking in a stately procession through the hurly-burly of the London streets, dressed in their distinctive purple robes, the college censors, along with the wardens and beadles of the Society of Apothecaries, would move from shop to shop. Once inside, Harvey examined the medicines and threw any adulterated powders he found out of the front door into the street. There they grew into a multicoloured molehill, while the apothecary helplessly looked on. Harvey soon discovered all the tricks of the fraudulent apothecaries' trade: how they thinned down diascordium (an electuary recommended by Galen) with honey; how they made up Gascoin's powder (prescribed for measles and smallpox) without including the more expensive ingredients.

Harvey was so appalled by such double-dealing that he peti-

tioned the king for stricter rules and severer fines for any apothecary found guilty of a misdemeanour. Representing
the college before King James' Privy Council, he implored the
body to promulgate a law ensuring that no apothecary could
'make medecyne without a living Doctor's bill . . . Any
one doing otherwise', should, he argued 'be punished by law
as a public enemy against the life of man.' When his request
was granted, Harvey was given the unenviable task of
explaining to the Society of Apothecaries 'the justnes of the
demaunds made by the College' and of 'persuading them to
Conformitye'.

At his meeting with the Privy Council, Harvey also requested
that a law be passed 'concerning Chirurgions [surgeons], that they
shall not doe any great operation in Chirurgerye without calling a
Doctor to Counsell'. To further their cause, Harvey lobbied
Parliament, pleading with the Members for Cambridge to support
the college against the surgeons. After a prolonged struggle, the
college prevailed. They had been very astute in their selection of
Harvey as spokesmen for their campaign, recognizing in him leader-
ship qualities typical of choleric men, such as tenacity, diligence,
and ruthlessness.

The apothecaries and surgeons avenged their defeat by casting
aspersions on the physicians, informing potential patients that the
college was only interested in power and money, and negligent of
its offices. As physicians' fees were exorbitant, and as their track
record did not inspire great confidence, these attacks were often
effective, with many patients choosing to consult apothecaries,
surgeons or empirics, rather than call on fellows of the college. The
majority of people, however, had little faith in the medical profession generally, and would attempt to heal themselves by appealing
to God, or by allowing nature to take its course, before consulting
anyone.

On 25 February 1609 Harvey left his house and walked west under Ludgate, built into the Roman wall that encircled the city. He then turned north into Olde Baily, proceeded up Gifford Street, until he arrived at Smithfield, site of one of London's largest cattle, pig, sheep and horse markets. Smithfield was notorious for its shabbiness: the poor of the area hung their 'beddings and bestly rags before their doors', emptied 'foul vessels' and 'washed animals' in the streets. Harvey is likely to have raised his luxurious purple gown as he walked, to prevent it from trailing in the puddles and refuse. 'London', the country boy lamented, 'is full of the filth of men, animals, sewers, and other forms of squalor.'

Harvey then walked east towards the spire of St Bartholomew the Less, the parish church of St Bartholomew's Hospital, his destination. It was London's oldest hospital, having been founded by the monk Rahere in 1123, 'to wait upon the sick' of the city 'with all diligence and care'. Harvey passed under the hospital's baroque stone gate, decorated with stained-glass windows, and a large round clock.

The hospital governors awaited Harvey in the Great Hall, which he reached after passing through a maze of courts, neat gardens, passageways and arches. After introducing himself to the governors, Harvey showed them a testimony of his skills from the president and senior doctors of the College of Physicians. 'I am making sute', he explained, 'for the office of hospital physician in reversion'—which was to say when it would be next vacant. Harvey then produced letters of recommendation from the king, which he may have obtained through the college, and, particularly, through friends of his father-in-law. After reading the documents the governors granted Harvey's request, making him assistant to the current physician, Dr Wilkinson, with immediate effect. When Wilkinson died six months later, Harvey was admitted to the office of physician.

St Bartholomew's was one of the two great London hospitals which catered for the sick poor. There were twelve wards, containing over 200 beds, covered with multicoloured blankets.

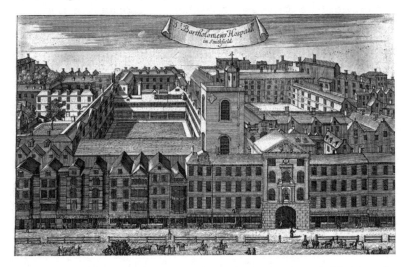

St Bartholomew's Hospital (1720). The vast complex extended south as far as Greyfriars Church, and encompassed large private houses and gardens.

The indigent sick pleaded for admittance at the gate, or they were rounded up by hospital beadles who were instructed by the governors to scour the city for anyone with a 'loathly grief or disease' lying 'open in any notable place, to the annoyance and infection of the passer-by'. Having identified a patient, the beadles ordered an almoner to convey him to the hospital, on a stretcher if need be.

The patients were tended to by twelve sisters, who were supervised by the matron, the chief governess of the house. The medical staff consisted of the physician, the apothecaries and the surgeons.

During his time in office, Harvey drew up strict rules defining the roles and relative importance of the staff. No surgeon was to give 'inward physic to the poor without the approbation of the Doctor'; every surgeon should 'follow the directions of the Doctor in outward operations for inward causes for the recovery of every patient under their several cures'. To that end, the surgeons, along with the apothecaries, should 'attend the Doctor at a set hour to [hear his] directions'.

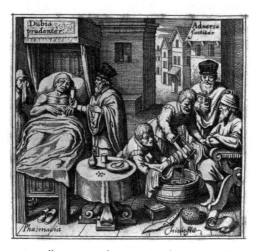

Seventeenth-century illustration showing apothecaries and surgeons tending to their patients. At St Bartholomew's the surgeons performed operations on inmates in the ward.

This consultation took place in the Great Hall, where Harvey presided at least once a week. This was in accordance with the 'Charge of the Physician' which commanded him to 'come to this Hospitall, and cause the Matron to call before you in the hall such and soe many of the poore as shall neede counsel & advise. And you are required & desired, in God his most holy name, that you endevour yourselfe to doe the beste of your knowledge [for them].'

The arthritic, the apoplectic, the paralysed, the pox-ridden, the jaundiced and the syphilitic were brought up one by one by the sisters, sometimes on stretchers, to the thirty-one-year-old Harvey who sat enthroned in the Great Hall, in his purple cap and robes. Drawing close to the patient, Harvey would gain their confidence by his courteous manner, listening carefully as they described their ailment. He then took the patient's pulse, not timing it but feeling for its strength or faintness, and examined a sample of their fresh urine. Harvey smelt the contents of the glass, then held the liquid up to the light, to see if it were cloudy or whether there was any sediment floating within it. 'What says the doctor to my water?' the bolder patients might ask.

If Harvey decided that a medicine would help a patient, he gave his instructions to the attending apothecaries, who would 'wryte in a booke appointed for that purpose, such medicines with theire compounds and necessaries, to be provyded and made reddy for to be ministred'. If he favoured external treatment, Harvey would call one of the surgeons and give him detailed orders as to how to proceed.

After closely examining a patient crippled by rheumatic pains, Harvey would ask both the apothecaries and the surgeons to lend him their ears. He explained to them that the man should:

> first take a clyster [enema] about fore of the clock in the afternoone . . . The next day about eight or nine of the clock let him bleed out of the arme eight or nine ounce of blood; afterwards continue to take his Apozem [infusion] twice in the day . . . and walke abroad and use moderate exercise . . . After he hath continued in this course of clearing his body 14 or 15 dayes let him every morning before he arise out of his bed have his belly and sides rubbed . . . All this while he taketh this physicke let his dyet bee temperate, of one dish, [let him] rise early, abstaine from wine, strong drinke and all salt meates.

Harvey's instructions were conventional. Steeped in Galenic medicine, he believed that the four humours within the body had to be carefully regulated, imbalance being the cause of most illness. Harmony and health could be re-established within the patient's body by purging, bloodletting, dieting or medicine, to be employed in a variety of combinations. Purging by emetics and bloodletting were the commonest medical remedies: 'all patients', one eminent physician declared, 'were the better for evacuants in the early stages of disease, whatever the condition'; another adopted as his motto 'Always let blood in cases of great distress until the patient faints.'

Such treatments (along with better living conditions) assisted the recovery of some 400 patients per year. When an inmate was deemed well enough to be discharged, he was presented to the physician in the Great Hall. Kneeling down in front of Harvey's throne the patient waited for the physician to pronounce him cured, then gave praise to God and to the hospital's staff. Before leaving the institution, he was provided with money, clothes, and a passport with which he could travel, unmolested by the authorities, to family or friends—if he were lucky enough to possess any.

7. Advances (c.1610–c.1625): 'Good endeavours bring forth much good frute'

THE WEALTHY CITY merchant Sir William Smith had been suffering for months from a large stone in his bladder. Although the pain was excruciating he was loath to be 'cut for the stone', an extremely dangerous and painful operation, during which the surgeon made an incision near the base of the penis, then groped around inside the bladder with a tool called a ducks bill. 'If the stone be greater than may be drawne forth at the hole', a diarist wrote, 'the partie dyes for it.' Desperate with fear, Sir William summoned Harvey to his London home.

During the initial consultation, the physician inserted his finger into his patient's rectum in order to feel for the stone. What Harvey discovered gave him hope. The stone was so tiny that an operation would not be necessary. 'Have patience for a month', he counselled, 'for I have a secret [medicine] which no man in England has but me, and I will make trial of it and do not doubt that it will do you much good and even dissolve the stone.' 'Good doctor,' an ecstatic Sir William replied, 'let me have the medicine and let my apothecary make it because he knoweth the state of my body best.' 'No', Harvey, responded, 'I shall make it up myself; for I am desirous that no man but myself learn the ingredients.' Jubilant at the prospect of a painless cure, Smith offered Harvey an annuity of

£50, to be paid in quarterly amounts of £12.10s., for as long as he did not have to be cut for the stone.

If Harvey was wary of calling upon Sir William's surgeon to perform an operation, and suspicious of his apothecary, he was openly hostile to the merchant's resident doctor, the empiric John Emerson, a vicar from Shoreham. On encountering the unqualified physician in Sir William's bedchamber, the choleric doctor ordered the 'horse leech' to return to his provincial parish; invoking the authority of the College of Physicians he 'did also threaten to lay him in prison for his meddling in what therein he had no skill'. Emerson countered by boasting of his success in curing countless 'knights and ladies'; Sir William also rallied to his defence. 'If you imprison any man that shall want to do me good Doctor Harvey, I will quickly find means to enlarge him again.' Knowing that it would be foolish to challenge a knight of the realm, the physician was forced to retreat.

Harvey administered to Sir William the miracle medicine, recommending a 'very stict and sparing diet' for the duration of the cure. He visited Sir William regularly, and was sanguine in his prognosis. 'Your water is better than it was', he would announce cheerfully, 'I can keep you at this stage [dosage]'. Yet the patient perceived no improvement in his condition; indeed his agony only intensified with every passing day.

During one visit Sir William announced 'I tell you plainly that (when all is done) I must be cut for, because I am not able to be so tortured as I am; my pains are so great as that they will distract me from my senses.' Harvey counselled patience, but Sir William feared his suffering would cause him to lose his mind: 'it is not possible for me to live in this manner as I do, so by God's grace I will adventure it [the operation]'. Harvey reluctantly agreed to call for the surgeon. 'If you be cut', he added, making reference to their financial arrangement, 'I do not intend to demand [further payment] of you'—though he still wished to be paid for the time he had tended upon Sir William up to the operation.

Sir William's surgeon successfully removed a huge stone from his bladder. But a urinary infection ensued soon afterwards, contaminating his kidneys. Within two months, Sir William was dead. On his deathbed he mustered up the energy to curse his physician, and expressly commanded his son 'not to pay Harvey' the £12 10s still owed on his annuity. Harvey was determined, however, to obtain the outstanding fee, and brought a common law action against the family.

This was not an isolated instance of unsound judgement on Harvey's part. Surgeons often accused him of erroneously (and self-interestedly) prescribing medicine in cases where external treatment was necessary, thus causing patients to die 'by ill practice'. A fellow doctor claimed that one of Harvey's medicines sent a patient instantaneously to 'the Close Stool' and from thence almost as rapidly to 'the other world'. A friend of Harvey's confirmed that he 'never heard of any [physician] that admired [Harvey's] Therapeutique way. I knew several practitioners that would not have given 3d for one of his Bills; and [who said] that a man could hardly tell by one of his Bills what he did aime at.'

In the highly competitive and litigious world of medicine, accusations of malpractice were common. Yet even some of Harvey's patients complained that his diagnoses were fanciful and inaccurate. One characterized him as an indifferent and uncaring doctor 'yet he pretends very much to study and lay my case to heart'.

Despite his mixed reputation as a physician, Harvey's private practice flourished. Through his contacts at the College of Physicians he had access to noble men and women willing to pay dearly for his services. Poor lame Sir Davy Gam sought his advice; Sir Thomas Hardes consulted him about his urethral stricture. Such patients dwelt in the penumbra of King James I's presence, on the outer circles of the court, and they may have afforded Harvey partial access to it. It was perhaps on their recommendation that the Lord Treasurer consulted Harvey during an attack of urinary calculus.

William's brother John, the second of the seven Harvey boys, and some four years his younger, also offered him an entrée to the court. Settling in London, presumably soon after his older brother, John had ingratiated himself at court, eventually becoming 'one of his majesty's footmen'. When or how John secured the position is unknown, but his good fortune was not unusual; the Scots king often favoured men of lowly backgrounds, much to the chagrin of men of aristocratic status who complained of a court crammed full of 'scum such as . . . sheep-reeves, yeomen's sons, pedlar's sons'. From the lowly position of footman John rose to the rank of 'yeoman of the bedchamber', performing his duties in a magnificent livery of ruff and doublet embellished with the Tudor rose. John had the unenviable task of dressing the notoriously slovenly king, yet he was rewarded with wages of around £50 a year, and by the influence he could now exert on behalf of friends and family. It is just possible that it was through John that William had obtained the letters of recommendation from the king, with which he secured his post at St Bartholomew's.

Court was the epicentre of power and influence. The grants, pensions, monopolies and positions on offer there made it a magnet for the ambitious. James was infamous for auctioning off titles and sinecures in return for much-needed cash, having failed to secure an income through either Parliament, taxation, or forced loans from his subjects. The court was a motley gaggle of 1,500 members, comprised of preachers and players, physicians and musicians, who followed the king's wandering progress between his London residences at the Tower, Whitehall, Bridewell Palace and Hampton Court. Days passed in a round of gossiping, diplomacy, scheming and feasting; meals and entertainments were lavish.

Having entered this labyrinth of potential patients and contacts, Harvey now had to navigate his way successfully. It is difficult, perhaps, to imagine the lowly and intensely intellectual country boy mastering, in the full glare of the court, the art of plucking off his napkin gracefully, footing it with dancing, warbling along when a general song was carolled up, or chatting away chivalrously to the ladies. Despite his Italian sojourn he may have lacked the elegance, poise and *sprezzatura* for such refined capering and carousing. Harvey would probably have had little natural inclination, either, to keep up with all the court news—'who loses and who wins, who's in, who's out'.

Yet if Harvey's first steps at court were hesitant and awkward, soon enough he was sauntering, if not exactly swaggering, his way through it. He seems to have learned quickly enough how to 'flatter and look fair'. In the portrait painted of him in the 1620s, he wears a fashionable puce-coloured fustian doublet and a velvet mantle and ruff.

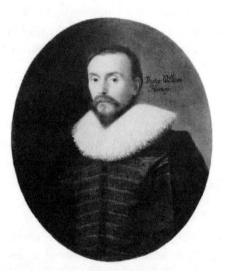

There is something aloof and detached about Harvey's expression in this 1620s portrait: while he seems proud of being a courtier, it is as though he is merely *posing* as one.

Harvey's everyday attire was elegant too, consisting of a rich black cloak, full doublet, ribbed stocking of black silk, and long high-heeled boots fringed at the top. When visiting patients Harvey decked himself out in his purple robe; on his journey to their homes he always 'rode on horseback with a footcloath . . . his man following on foote', which was reckoned very decent, and the height of fashion.

The yeoman's son also developed great fluency in polite discourse. 'My sweete Lord,' he would write in letters to gentlemen, 'yf ever I have done and may be able to doe service to you ther is nothing wilbe more comfort and joy unto me, wheare all good endeavours bring forth much good frute and all service is soe plentifully acknowledged.'

With the right contacts, and the appropriate doublet and conversation, Harvey eventually came to the notice of King James himself, being appointed one of his 'physicians extraordinary' in 1618. The king, who was regarded by many as ineffectual, wilful and overly fond of his own coarse jokes, would nevertheless have been interesting to Harvey from a medical point of view, his constitution being extremely susceptible to disturbances.

> The King's mind is moved suddenly. He is very wrathful, but the fit soon passes off. Sometimes he is melancholy from the spleen [which] . . . easily heaps up melancholic juice . . . Urine generally normal. Impatient of sweat as of all things . . . After [a] great sadness [he experiences] diarrhoea for eight days . . . fainting, sighing, dread, intermittent pulse . . . there [has been] a descent of humours into his right arm whence arose swollen glands.

King James would have been a difficult patient for Harvey, owing to these manifold complaints, which were compounded by his volatility and lack of fortitude. 'He is of extreme sensitiveness, impatient of pains', wrote one of Harvey's colleagues, 'and while they torture him with most violent movements, his mind is tossed and bile flows.' To make matters worse, James, like so many of his contemporaries, had no confidence whatsoever in the opinion of his physicians. 'The King laughs at medicine and holds it so cheap that he declares physicians to be hardly necessary. He asserts the art to be supported by mere conjectures and useless because uncertain.'

In 1625 Harvey followed a melancholy king to Theobalds, his Hertfordshire retreat. First crippled by an ague, then felled by a sudden stroke, the king was finally overwhelmed by a violent attack of dysentery 'dangerous unto death', and took to his bed. Harvey administered to his needs tirelessly but to little effect. He could see that the 'former Vigour of Nature' was 'low and spent' in his master. Knowing that his end was approaching, James asked his chaplain to 'make me ready to go away to Christ'. After prayers were intoned over him, James raised his hands up to his face and shut his own eyes.

Soon after James' son Charles ascended the throne he awarded Harvey the sum of £100 'as of His Majesty's free gift, for his pains and attendance about the person of His Majesty's late dear father, of happy memory, in time of his sickness'. Charles I also retained Harvey as a physician extraordinary, in time promoting him to physician in ordinary—a far more important position, which carried with it an annual salary of £300, a pension of £400 per annum, and a daily 'diet of three dishes of meat a meal, with all incidents thereunto belonging'.

Harvey's official duties included prescribing medicine for the royal household, tending upon its members during bouts of illness, and accompanying them, or their favourites, on their travels abroad. This left him little time for his commitments to either the College of Physicians or St Bartholomew's Hospital, but he was excused from these, the king having the precedent claim.

The fastidious and forbidding Charles was far less approachable than his father. The new king insisted on formality at all times, never allowing a visitor to be seated in his or his queen's presence. But however aloof he was with other members of his court, Charles enjoyed conversing relatively freely with Harvey, with whom he shared a number of intellectual interests.

Harvey and the king discussed medicine, natural philosophy and the physiology of the numerous animals belonging to the Crown.

Sometimes Harvey would crave an audience with Charles, in order to show him a 'pretty Spectacle and Rarity of Nature'. On one occasion he brought a petrified child's skull, excavated in Crete, into the royal presence; His Majesty 'wondered at it & looked content to see so rare a thing'.

Harvey professed to value learning over titles. 'When he perceived', a friend said, 'that honours and other decorations of that kind' were not, in the main, given as rewards for 'uprightness of character' or 'dedication to philosophy', he 'passed all these things by'— meaning perhaps, that he never petitioned the king for a knighthood. Harvey did not, it seems, covet a title; being the king's personal physician, and one of his resident intellectuals, was apparently satisfaction enough.

The doctor was certainly satisfied with the wealth that accompanied his meteoric rise through the social and professional ranks. His unconcealed enthusiasm for money may have been frowned on at court. Self-interest was no more an aristocratic virtue than it was a Christian one, the principal value of money, according to aristocrats, being that it enabled one to improve the commonwealth, by helping the poor, or furthering diplomatic and religious causes. Yeomen such as Harvey believed, however, that they might justly enrich themselves as it was their only means of climbing the social ladder.

Harvey methodically accrued a considerable fortune through his services to the Crown and his lucrative private practice. As a physician he drove a very hard bargain, and insisted his patients stuck to it. He often pursued outstanding payments via the courts, even when the legal costs added up to far more than the fees in question. For Harvey there was doubtless a principle at stake—his right to be paid a fee for a service rendered.

Thomas Harvey may have instilled this principle in his eldest son, along with other yeoman values. Yeomen were supposed to live with the utmost temperance and thrift. Although he enjoyed dressing the part of the courtier physician, Harvey's 'tastes in food, and other necessities of life' were, a friend said, always of the simplest kind. Like the rest of his family too he was renowned for tight-fistedness.

Harvey ensured that his money did not, in the words of another shrewd yeoman of the period, 'lye idly by hym'; instead, according to a contemporary biographer, 'as soon as he had gathered together any [sum] of value he either bought property therewith or put the same out to Interest'. He purchased from one William Lodges of Gray's Inn a 'new brick tenement lying in a street called Hart street in Covent Garden' which he presumably rented out. He also acquired 'fifty-nine acres of land in the Parish of Petham Kent' from Thomas Court of Waltham. And when the time was ripe, Harvey sold on his purchases. William Laud, the Archbishop of Canterbury, and one of King Charles' trusted counsellors, purchased from the physician and his brothers the 'vicarage rectory & parsonage' that were formerly part of 'ye late Priory of Folkestone', indicating that Harvey speculated in property that had formerly been sacred.*

In all these dealings Harvey was assisted by his father. Thomas, along with his six other sons, had moved up to Hackney in London from Kent, some years after his wife's death in 1605. All of the Harvey boys prospered in the capital, under the watchful eye of their father. While John advanced at court, the others (Thomas, Daniel, Eliab, Matthew and Michael), having been apprenticed in trade, now made fortunes as merchants of goods from the Levant and Far East. All of the boys made their father the treasurer of

---

* The full extent of Harvey's land and property portfolio only came to light in 2001, when a wrought iron Armada chest, adorned with flowers and allegorical figures, and dating from around 1600, was discovered. Various descendants of the Harvey family appear to have placed documents relating to their forebears within the chest, and shut them up in around 1820 to lay undisturbed there for almost two centuries.

their lands, as their wily old 'pinchfart penny-father' (as parsimo-
nious patriarchs were known) was 'as skilful to purchase Land as
they to gain Money; and he kept, employed, and improved their
farmings to their great advantage'.

Thomas exhorted his sons to 'live in the fear . . . of Almighty
God and unite with one another fast knit together, as [you] may
be evermore a helpe one to another'. They followed this command
assiduously, each assisting the others with advice, favours and
money. The yeoman patriarch must have delighted in watching
their collective ascent to wealth, 'seeing the meanest of them of
far greater estate than himself' being one of his two great
ambitions.

Sometime after 1614 Thomas set about realizing his other
dream—achieving the status of gentleman. He applied to the Garter
King of Arms for permission to bear a coat of arms, an honour
only conferred (officially at least) on those 'whose race and blood
or virtues do make noble and knowne'—that is to say, men of
distinguished pedigree, or those whose families had performed great
services to Crown and country. In reality, it was often simply a
question of hard cash. Prospective gentlemen had to prove that
they possessed a fortune of several hundred pounds, dressed well,
kept servants, and were wealthy enough to bribe the relevant
officials. Men of gentle birth often complained of the corruption
which made it possible for yeomen, such as 'Shakespeare ye player',
to qualify as gentlemen.

Having satisfied the Garter King of Arms of his fortune (while
spuriously claiming, for good measure, descent from the thirteenth-
century Mayor of London, Sir Walter Harvey) Thomas was allowed
to present a pattern for his coat of arms to the College of Heralds.
The shield contained silver crescents, the emblem of Levant
merchants, a testament perhaps to Thomas' intimate involvement
with his sons' commercial ventures. When the design was approved,
the yeoman born became a made gentleman and so did his male
descendants.

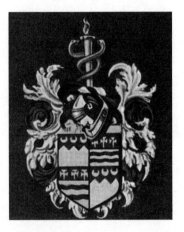

A version of the Harvey coat of arms, which can be seen on several post-humous portraits of William Harvey, evidencing the family's pride in having secured gentlemanly status.

A weary but doubtless satisfied Thomas passed away in 1623, in his mid-seventies, escutcheons with the Harvey coat of arms proudly adorning his coffin. Displaying no trace of sentimentality, William decided to perform the autopsy on his father's body himself, Thomas encouraging his son's medical studies in death as well as in life. Harvey was rewarded by the opportunity of examining his father's exceptionally 'huge' colon, an anatomical curiosity which he would refer to in his public lectures.

PART II:
PLACING HIS HEAD AMONG THE STARS

8. A public lecture (late 1610s): 'Nasty (yet recompensed by admirable variety)'

I<small>N</small> 1615 <small>THE</small> College of Physicians appointed the thirty-seven-year-old William Harvey as Lumleian lecturer in anatomy for life. The position brought him considerable cachet as the public and intellectual face of the college; it also offered a very welcome stipend. Officially the anatomical lectures (first instituted in 1582 by Lord Lumley) were to be delivered for 'three quarters of an hour in Latine, and [one] quarter of an hour in English, wherin that shall be plainlie declared for those that understand not Latine, what was said in Latine'.

In preparation for his lectures, Harvey compiled copious Latin notes. His jottings also contain numerous remarks in English, the language he often employed when offering an illustration of a general statement. In this characteristically vivid and homely quotation, for example, the words in italics were originally written in English, the rest in Latin: 'Examples of motion . . . *hawke putts over her meate crap turning upon the giserd erecte itself*. Likewise *a dog: by the fier: cunny in ye sunn.*'

Harvey may in fact have departed from the college statutes and given his lectures mostly in the vernacular, using his Latin notes as a guide, summarizing and translating them as he went along, rather than reading from them verbatim. The members of the

A page from Harvey's lecture notes. Fragmentary, cryptic and elliptical, they were compiled, altered and augmented over the period c.1615–1629.

Barber Surgeons Company, at whom the lectures were principally aimed, were ignorant of Latin, not having been educated at university. Barbers had been the first surgeons in England, originally assisting monks, who were forbidden for religious reasons from performing operations. The Barbers Company had been founded in 1462, the surgeons amalgamating with them a century later. By the turn of the seventeenth century surgeons performed most operations, but barbers still carried out bloodletting—hence the red and white barber's pole that was the emblem of their trade, the red signifying blood, the white the cloth of the tourniquet.

Every year of his lectureship Harvey had to offer a course on 'the whole art of anatomy', over a five-day period, 'dissecting all the body of [a single] man, if the body may so last without annoie'. In a bid to preserve the corpse for as long as possible, dissections took place in winter, yet despite that decomposition was usually so rapid that a number of bodies had to be cut up over the course. Generally, one corpse was dissected during the muscular lecture to show the muscles, another to display the bones in the osteological lecture, with a third for the visceral lecture, during which the abdomen, the thorax and then the head were anatomized in turn. The visceral lecture especially had to be conducted, in Harvey's phrase, 'according to the glass' (i.e. with a close eye on the hourglass): the abdomen came first because it decayed most rapidly, being crammed full of matter that was 'nasty (yet recompensed by admirable variety)'. Then came the thorax ('the parlour' of the body), because it decomposed next, and last of all came the more durable brain.

In his lectures Harvey aimed to show, in the words of his notes, the 'action, function and purpose of the parts', to investigate morbid conditions, and to present 'problems in the authors'—that is, controversies in the anatomical tradition. He also offered a comprehensive course in 'the whole art' of surgery and dissection for the barbers and surgeons, promising to 'cut up as much as may be, so that the skill [in cutting] may illustrate the narrative'. In addition, he endeavoured to 'show as much in one observation as can be', and 'not to speak of anything which without the carcase may be delivered or read at home'. Although he would introduce some Aristotelian elements into his lectures (using animal carcasses occasionally, in the manner of Fabricius, and perhaps even performing experiments on live animals) Harvey generally adopted the hands-on, human body-centred anatomical style of Vesalius. The style was tailored to his audience, the barbers and surgeons requiring practical instruction, and the physicians, steeped in Galenic anatomy, being exclusively interested in human physiology and pathology.

Harvey lectures were performed at five o'clock sharp at the anatomy theatre in the College of Physicians' magnificent three-storeyed premises at Amen Corner, to which it had migrated from Knight Ryder Street in 1614. Here, on a winter's evening in the late 1610s, the entire body of the Barber Surgeons gathered for a lecture, dressed in their black gowns and flat caps. Members of the college were in evidence too, seating themselves towards the front of the audience, attired in wool or silk. Several courtiers sat down with them, along with various gentlemen and law students.* The hall's hearth was fireless, the breath of the audience visible in the nipping air.

The lecturer and the dissection table were hidden from the audience's view behind a circular curtain. In accordance with the college statutes, a mat had been placed next to the table so that Harvey did not 'take colde upon his feet'. A sixteen-inch whalebone wand with a silver tip lay on the table so that the lecturer might 'touche the body when it shall please him'. There was a candle with which he could 'loke into the bodye', as well as an assortment of surgical instruments. Next to these lay a number of bowls and sponges. Finally, there was the body of the recently hanged man, which had been washed, shaven and hollowed out at the abdomen, which resembled a pink, bloody cave. Harvey had eviscerated it the previous evening; tonight it was the turn of the thorax.

* In 1662, the ever busy, ever curious Samuel Pepys, clerk of the king's ships, would find time to attend an anatomy at the Barber Surgeons, performed by one of Harvey's disciples. Pepys enjoyed a 'fine good discourse' on the mysteries of the body, the subject on the occasion being a 'lusty fellow, a seaman, hanged for robbery'. The civic and legal aspect of the dissection was made explicit, with the audience being informed of the subject's occupation, crime and punishment.

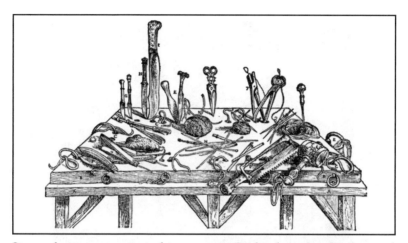

Sixteenth-century anatomical instruments. For his dissections Harvey used knives, probes, lancets, hooks, drills, razors, scalpels and dilators, some of which can be seen here.

Behind the curtain the stewards dressed Harvey in a white bonnet and a gleaming white apron with detachable sleeves covering 'the whole arm with tapes for chaunge'. As it was 'unseemly' for an anatomist to 'occupy one aprone and one payr of sleves' for the whole of the messy and bloody five-day demonstration, the stewards prepared a fresh set each day. An additional apron and pair of sleeves lay beside the dissection table, in case the first set became too soiled during the lecture.

On the stroke of five, the stewards drew back the curtain and the spectators reacquainted themselves with the bruised cadaver. Those in the front rows caught on the air the pungent odour of the decaying flesh. Sometimes the demonstration conformed to the conventional anatomical model, with Harvey reading his lecture while an *ostensor-cum-sector* (usually a barber) carried out the cutting. On occasion, however, Harvey followed Vesalius in cutting the corpse himself, and we may picture him doing so on this particular evening. A barber, also dressed in white, stood by the table, on hand to assist him.

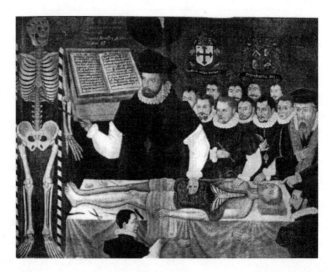

John Banister giving a lecture on the abdomen to surgeons and barbers in 1581. He is describing the bone structure displayed by the skeleton; an anatomical text rests on the lectern behind him.

Harvey set about opening up the thorax of the corpse with a knife, describing in considerable detail the incisions he made as he went along. 'Now with a sharp knife, I will set about freeing the clavicle [collarbone] from the sternum [breastbone] dividing the strong ligaments. See how I take care lest the knife be driven too deeply and injure the vessels lying beneath.' Harvey made the incisions, his assistant hovering around the body with a sponge to wipe away any blood that seeped out of the openings.

'Forcibly', he went on, 'I then raise the freed cartilages and bend the first rib outward from the sternum . . . the cartilage must be freed from the rib with a razor.' Harvey bent back the first rib and put his knife down on the table, where it was wiped by the assistant. He then took up a razor, using it to cut the cartilage away from the rib. 'And now I will do the same with all of the other ribs in turn.' The task took Harvey and his assistant some time to complete. When all of the ribs had been raised and cleaned, Harvey took up his knife again and divided the intercostal muscles with a continuous incision as far down as the base of the thorax.

Quick, decisive and supremely confident, Harvey's handiwork excited the admiration of the audience. Although not yet forty, the small, round-shouldered anatomist was already the veteran of numerous public anatomies and countless private autopsies. The authority he displayed during lectures earned him the reputation of a consummate performer. One spectator would praise, in a series of Latin verses, Harvey's 'marvellous dissecting', 'clever hand' and 'dexterity beyond compare'. Brandishing the scalpel as adroitly as Hercules 'wielded his club', the Englishman was 'unrivalled at the table'.

Harvey now required all his strength, as well as all his dexterity, as he attempted to free the man's breastbone from his ribs. 'The sternum must be bent somewhat upward and then to the right and left, toward the head'; with these words he removed the breastbone with its vessels from the thorax. Using a hook he 'pulled away here and there the membrane lining the ribs', then, with his hands, he separated the membrane from the lung before attempting to break the ribs 'almost in their middle'. Harvey accomplished this by 'grasping firmly with the hands and twisting and bending forcibly', his assistant again coming to his aid.

The work of removal complete, the heart (which would be the focus of this lecture) was now laid bare. With a knife Harvey cleaned away the fat surrounding it. He then held up a lit candle to the exposed thorax, so that the spectators could see the organ clearly. 'The heart', he announced, 'is situated at the fourth and fifth ribs, in the very middle of the body. It is the principal organ because it is in the principal place. In quantity the heart of man is, as you see, fairly large. The substance of the heart'—here he prodded the man's heart with the silver tip of the whalebone rod—'is dense, thick, hard flesh, compacted like the kidneys. We can say that the temperament of the heart is very hot, since it is very full of blood.'

Harvey indicated the various parts of the heart to the audience. He first pointed out the vena cava, which brought blood from the veins to the right side of the heart. With the rod he traced the transit of the vena cava through the thorax, and its 'distribution in the root of the neck'. He then grasped the heart in his hands, and, squeezing the organ, indicated the pulmonary artery on the right side near to the vena cava. 'It is whitish', he said, and 'is the highest of the vessels of the heart.' Its function was to carry blood from the right side of the heart down into the lungs.

Turning to the left side of the heart Harvey pointed out the pulmonary vein, 'which coveys blood from the lungs to the left side of the heart; it is darker than the pulmonary artery'. Then he turned to the aorta, 'the great artery', which 'carries vivified blood throughout the body. It is near the entrance of the pulmonary vein.'

Harvey made an incision in the right side of the heart with a razor. He then squeezed the right ventricle with his fingers so that the purple blood inside it oozed out, his assistant wiping this away with a sponge. Harvey indicated the inside of the vena cava, opening it up further with a stylus. Inserting a long, thick rod into it, he then showed the audience how it extended down to the lower reaches of the body. Moving on to the pulmonary artery he put his finger into its orifice, located in the higher part of the right side of the heart, his assistant again mopping up the blood that issued out of it. Next he 'followed the course of the pulmonary artery, into the lungs' with his rod. Having finished with the right side of the heart, Harvey then cut the left ventricle in the same fashion, and proceeded to display to the audience the interior of the pulmonary vein, and the aorta, with the help of a stylus and a knife.

In his lectures, Harvey generally offered a synopsis of conventional theory. He was reluctant to draw extensively on his own opinions, nor did he 'disprayse' other anatomists, but rather expressed the conservative view that all his anatomical predecessors 'had done well', those found to be culpable of error being so solely because of chance. Harvey frequently complimented the 'great' Galen, explaining away the discrepancies between the Greek's theories and the dissected body on the table by suggesting that the human body itself had altered since Roman times. It was diplomatic of Harvey to excuse Galen in front of his fellow physicians whose medical therapies and authority were underpinned by Galenic theories. In compiling his lecture notes Harvey had used as a crib Caspar Bauhin's orthodox anatomical manual, *Theatrum anatomicum* (1605).

Yet there were times when the Lumleian lecturer's language became more idiosyncratic, occasions when he introduced a note of doubt into his summaries of received opinion. Scattered throughout his fragmentary lecture notes is a personal shorthand that served as a commentary on the conventional text. The symbol 'X' prompted Harvey to offer a concrete illustration of whatever he happened to be discussing; it also served as a cue for him to air disagreement with a particular theory. The letters 'WH' (William Harvey) indicated an opportunity to furnish his listeners with an original observation or example.

In describing the movement of blood, within the arteries and veins that carried it throughout the body, Harvey took the traditional line that it ebbed and flowed sluggishly in both directions. In discussing the muscular wall (septum) that divided the ventricles, however, he cast doubt on the validity of Galen's famous theory. Aware that Vesalius had questioned Galen's idea of the porous septum, Harvey treated the issue as a 'problem in the authors'—that is, as an anatomical controversy.

Pointing with his whalebone rod to the septum in front of him, Harvey declared: 'Galen believed that blood crosses the heart through the septum, through interstices in the wall; accordingly many hold the view that it is porous.' The symbol 'X' comes after the word 'porous' in Harvey's lecture notes, followed by the name 'Colombo'.

The Italian anatomist Realdo Colombo (c. 1515–1559) had been a pupil of Vesalius. Determined to surpass the mentor he referred to as a 'clumsy Belgian peasant' by any means fair or fowl (including plagiarism), Colombo set about rewriting various aspects of conventional anatomy. In discussing the septum in Book VII of *De re Anatomica* (*On Anatomy*)—a book which aimed to 'contradict all, both ancients and moderns'—Colombo had extended Vesalius' criticism of Galen. 'Between the ventricles of the heart', he remarked, 'is the septum, through which nearly everyone thinks that there is a way open for the blood to pass . . . But those who believe this err by a long way.' Contradicting Galen in such an emphatic manner would not have been welcomed by the physicians in Harvey's audience, so the lecturer doubtless trod carefully now as he retraced Colombo's footsteps. He may have watered down one of Colombo's bold pronouncements, alluding also perhaps to Vesalius' comments on the subject, and gently implying his own approval as he did so.

In his description of the vessels of the heart, Harvey had also drawn on Colombo's ideas, particularly when discussing the structure and role of the pulmonary artery and the pulmonary vein. The lecturer expanded upon his previous comments now. 'Blood is carried to the lung by the pulmonary vein', he quoted Colombo, 'and in the lung it is refined, and then together with the air it is brought through the pulmonary vein to the left ventricle of the heart.'

Colombo had posited this idea after observing, during numerous dissections, that the left side of the heart was always full of red arterial blood. The purple venous blood must, he concluded, travel from the right side of the heart to the lungs and, in doing so, became transformed there into 'shining' and 'beautiful' arterial blood. Galen had, he said, 'erroneously' located this transformation within the heart itself.

Although Harvey was citing an opinion that had not achieved the status of accepted truth, he was on relatively safe ground because Galen had also suggested that blood entered the lungs, albeit in a very small quantity and solely for the purpose of nourishing that organ.

Harvey then addressed the movement of the heart, another issue Colombo had recently made a 'problem in the authors'. The lecturer first explained to his audience the traditional Galenic view that the heart's active phase was expansion (known as diastole), the moment in which the organ was said to draw blood into itself from the veins. Some of the liquid then overflowed into the arteries, which also actively sucked blood out of the heart by virtue of a wave expansion (i.e. a pulse). The relaxing heart was then in a state of contraction, or systole. This, Galen maintained, was the *passive* phase of the heart's movement, 'concerned with death, and the internal rest of the heart after its forcible diastole.'

Harvey may have attempted to evoke the movements of the heart through the motion of his hands. He was a fine performer, with a repertoire of vivid gestures and the brio of an amateur actor, so it is easy to imagine him illustrating the pulsating organ. He may also have made other gestures for comic effect—when he described the 'waddle of a puffin', and the way ducks in motion 'sway this way and that', it is possible that he imitated the movements of these animals. He certainly enlivened his dissections with jokes whenever he could. Discussing callused skin, for instance, he used as an illustration the knees of overzealous Puritans who spent too long kneeling in prayer. Scatological references also abound: he described constipated men as all 'shite and groan' at stool.

Having presented Galen's theory of the movement of the heart,

Harvey turned to Colombo's opposing view. The Italian, Harvey explained, had argued that blood was forcefully ejected from the heart into the arteries when the organ contracted; systole was therefore its active phase, rather than diastole. If this was the case, Harvey continued, then the heart could be regarded as a muscle which moved like any other, in a cycle of contraction, relaxation and rest.

Colombo had arrived at his theory after performing countless vivisections on animals. Harvey probably mentioned these experiments to the audience, adding that he himself had likewise 'observed the movement of the heart in animals for whole hours at a time'. The announcement excited some surprise among the spectators, for vivisection was not commonly practised by English anatomists, nor was it of immediate relevance to the operations carried out by barbers and surgeons. It was also quite an audacious move for the lecturer to refer to his own experiments alongside those of acknowledged authorities. 'During those observations', Harvey went on boldly, 'I found it arduous and difficult, to discern what is systole and what diastole, for the heart in its running is always in motion. And yet it seems not unlikely to me that Colombo, rather than Galen, may have been closer to the truth about these matters.'

However interesting Harvey's discourse on the heart was, the barbers and surgeons could only absorb a certain amount of detail in a single sitting. Many became restless as they sat in the cold hall; some were doubtless relieved as Harvey brought the session to a close. The lecture was followed by a series of questions from the audience, during which Harvey was interrogated on his controversial comments regarding the septum, the movement of blood across the lungs and the movement of the heart.

The question and answer session over, the steward approached Harvey, took the whalebone rod from his hand, then turned to address the audience. 'This Lecture, Gentlemen, shall be continued tomorrow at five o'clock precisely.' The steward then invited the audience to follow him to the hall parlour, where a dinner had been prepared for them.

Colleagues approached Harvey to continue the discussion of the controversial points he had raised; the more curious students came up to the table to examine the dissected corpse closely, touching the body. Members of the general public also moved forward to look at the anatomized body, typically remarking on its 'unpleasantness', and 'appalling' smell. They were not alone in being offended by the stench of a carved-up cadaver: Harvey spoke of 'hands infected with the smell of carrion' after a dissection, and the overpowering smell of his 'sleeves during an anatomy'. Around four hours after an anatomy, he said, such smells seem to diminish, only to return again later with a vengeance.

Yet the sight and the smell of rotting flesh did not blunt the edge of the audience's appetite. The post-lecture dinner was a fine one, during which the king's health was enthusiastically toasted with beakers of wine. As they ate, the diners dissected the lecture. Sir Simon D'Ewes, a law student, sitting with some companions of his from the Middle Temple, reckoned he had gained 'much profitable knowledge'. Another spectator, who fancied himself as a poet, composed a verse eulogy to Harvey in which he 'rankt [him] among perui'. As 'perui' refers to the traditional venue for a formal disputation, the implication is that Harvey showed as much dexterity in argument as he did in cutting, being as skilled with 'knives as with words'.

Before the star performer joined his admirers at the dinner table, he and the stewards carefully examined the butchered corpse in the theatre to decide whether it was too putrid to be used again the following day. If it was rotten and another corpse was available, it could be dispensed with. In that case, the stewards would gather the remains together, place them in a coffin, and inter them at the expense of the college at a nearby church such as St Olave's, whose burial register contains references to a number of anatomized men and women. Inspection of the cadaver over, Harvey pulled off his robes and put on the clerk's gown that it was 'always usual for him to dine in'.

9. Private research (late 1610s–1620s): 'A dog, crow, kite, raven . . . anything to anatomize'

DURING THE 1610s and 1620s Harvey was busier than most of his colleagues, his professional life a ceaseless cycle of activity. The 'little perpetual mov[ement] Dr Heruye' examined patients at St Bartholomew's Hospital and often visited private clients in every corner of the city; he attended his lord and master the king as soon as he was summoned; he lectured, or transacted other official college business, at Amen Corner. Harvey's small feet and hands were always in motion, like the thoughts that raced around his head.

Having completed his numerous duties for the day, Harvey rode back to his black and white timber-framed Ludgate house. He might have been expected to pass most of his evenings at home pleasantly in the company of his wife, or with friends. Harvey was an amiable if not exactly gregarious man, and most physicians would have required leisure after the arduous labours of the day.

And yet it was often when Harvey returned home in the evenings that his real work—the work he pursued with all the obsessiveness of his ardent nature—began. Having entered his house, we may imagine him bidding his wife good evening, giving instructions to his servants, changing into his everyday black doublet, and then making his way to the chamber he had set aside for his private studies.*

On his way to the chamber, Harvey passed well-furnished rooms containing pictures, decorative hangings and chests full of linen. There was red damasked furniture in one of the rooms and a magnificent fireplace in another. Friends remarked on the simplicity of Harvey's taste and lifestyle, yet he was obliged to furnish his house as became a physician and a gentleman, because his colleagues, and some of his patients, visited him there. Sweet wax candles illuminated his home, rather than cheap 'stinking' tallow candles; he slept on 'gentleman's sheets' instead of the so-called 'yeoman's sheets' used by his servants.

Harvey's study contained a dissection table, on which his anatomical instruments lay. There was a clean white apron and a pair of gloves, left there by his servants, along with various anatomical books. Either within the chamber or more likely in an adjacent room, there was a vast menagerie of animals. Bottles and buckets containing toads, crabs, shrimps, whelks, oysters and fish of various kinds, lined the walls; there were lizards, tortoises, serpents, fowls, pigeons, geese, rabbits and mice scurrying around or lying lazily in cages and hutches. There may also have been larger kennels which accommodated Harvey's collection of clamorous sheep, pigs and dogs, although many of these animals were presumably kept in his garden or at a nearby stables. It was a private zoo, a Noah's ark of constant motion and confusion. On entering,

---

* Harvey was not the only natural philosopher of the period to dedicate a chamber in his house to private 'research', to use a modern term. It was not unknown for physicians to perform anatomies and autopsies in their private studies, or for those with alchemical interests to set up 'laboratories' there. Robert Hooke, the great experimenter of the later seventeenth century, used a dingy 'workshop-cellar' in his house, full of 'odd utensils and lumber'. Hooke's employer, the aristocrat Robert Boyle, constructed for himself a grand, temple-like 'laboratory' for his experiments, crammed full of marvellous devices, which was open to disciples and visitors.

Harvey examined the animals, selecting some as the subject of his investigations.

All of the animals found their way into Harvey's published writings, which also contain references to ants, dogfish, sharks, tadpoles, crocodiles, ostriches, emus, pheasants, wolves, horses, goats and elephants. It would, of course, have been impossible for Harvey to have kept, and experimented on, every one of these species at his Ludgate home—obtaining and housing an elephant in London would not have been easy. Some of his animal references are clearly to experiments and observations mentioned in books he read. Yet he undoubtedly examined the overwhelming majority of the animals he referred to.

Procuring 'mollusca unspecified, mussels, eels, barbell, tench, skate, stingrays, carp, herring, smelt, mullet' was easy enough for Harvey. The populous Thames gifted London fisherman 'trouts, breams, shrimps, herrings, eels, whiting, plaice, cods, mackerel' and 'sweet and fat salmons' by the ton. Fishwives sold them live in Fish Street Hill, Thames Street and Knyght Ryder Street: 'Turbot! All alive turbot!' they cried, 'Fish soles, oy, oy, alive! Alive, O!' Harvey also wandered down to the river at Blackfriars' Stairs, Powle's Wharf, Broken Wharf, and Queen Hithe, to examine the catches of the fishermen; vessels brimful of fish vied for the best position at these water gates.

Harvey was well known among the watermen of the Thames, and they kept the doctor abreast of curious occurrences. One day they told him of the Thames swallows who 'towards the end of the year, assemble in great numbers on the little islands of the river, and then submerge themselves within the water'; the men believed that they either turned into fish there or hibernated for the winter (the idea of bird migration was yet to be born). Harvey's curiosity was piqued. He asked the watermen to bring him some of the submerged birds. Dissecting them, he examined their insides for 'either warmth or motion' but found their organs to be lifeless and cold.

Harvey regularly visited the butchers' shops and slaughter-houses near Smithfield, to negotiate the purchase of warm-blooded animals and birds. For the horses, goats and sheep that prowled around his private zoo, he either went to Smithfield or had supplies sent up from family in Kent. On excursions outside the city he picked up everything and anything, living or dead, that happened to cross his path. Encountering a toad on a ramble he caught it up and stowed it away, or opened its belly there and then with a knife he always carried around with him. He often scoured the woods in search of 'a dog, crow, kite, raven or any bird, or anything to anatomize'. Harvey also had the free run of the royal parks, Charles granting him 'daily opportunity of dissecting' the buck and doe there, 'and of making inspection and observation of all their parts'. The king, Harvey boasted, 'much delighted in this kind of curiosity', and was 'many times pleased to be an eyewitness' at his physician's anatomies.

When Harvey compiled his Lumleian lecture notes in a notebook in the mid-1610s, he designed for them a title page on which he transcribed the following quotation from Aristotle: 'There is doubt about the internal parts of man, wherefore it is necessary to study in other animals those parts which bear a similarity to the parts of man.' The words were a proud declaration of faith—Harvey's private research would be Aristotelian. On the same page there was also a quotation from Virgil: 'I begin with Jove, O Muses. All things are filled with Jove.' This was a statement of Harvey's broader aim as a natural philosopher—to discern and reveal the hand of God working within His creation.

Fabricius had shown Harvey what an Aristotleian research programme might consist of. The Paduan professor had endeavoured to produce a complete description of every bodily organ, examining it in isolation and identifying its Aristotelian 'causes'. As those causes were displayed in diverse animal bodies, and as his definition of the organ had to be universally valid, Fabricius had cut up the carcasses of various animal species, including man.

Over the course of his illustrious career, Fabricius published the results of his investigations in volumes dedicated to the organs of 'vision', 'speech' and 'hearing'; he also wrote monographs on the 'respiration', 'generation' and 'motion' of animals, building directly on the researches of Aristotle himself in these areas. The Italian never realized his dream of producing an Aristotelian map of the entire body, yet he was acknowledged as a European authority on the areas he managed to cover.

Fabricius' approach seemed to Harvey to hold out the promise of yielding philosophically valid truth, as well as empirical knowledge, by combining inductive investigation based on the observation of the senses, and deductive Aristotelian reasoning. In his own work, Harvey solemnly vowed to 'tread in the footsteps of those who have lighted me the way; in chief, of all the *Ancients*, I follow *Aristotle*, and of the later Writers, *Hieronymous Fabricius ab Aquapendente*, Him as my general, and this as my guide.'

Harvey now resolved to replicate and if possible extend Fabricius' 'Aristotle project'. He was determined to bring Padua to London, to reconstruct the theatre of the Bo in his Ludgate home. Just like Linacre and Caius before him, Harvey would transplant the Italian revival of learning to England. It is not known exactly when, or precisely why, Harvey embarked on his research programme, at considerable expense to himself, but it must have been sometime after 1610 when he had fully established his medical practice and achieved a comfortable degree of wealth. His insatiable curiosity and extraordinary ambition obviously inspired his decision. The yeoman's son craved intellectual renown, now that he had secured social recognition. He dreamed of arriving at the point where he could boast that 'there was nothing in nature encompassed in so great obscurity or so recondite that he could not immediately unfold an explanation' of it.

As part of his research programme Harvey examined a set of

specific organs and body parts in isolation, analyzing their structure, purpose and function in as many animals as he could lay his hands on. In investigating the anus, he compared those of fowl such as geese and ducks to those of smaller birds such as the hedge sparrow, woodcock, thrush and blackbird; he then contrasted the anuses of these birds with those of fish such as the stingray.

Harvey followed in the footsteps of his mentors Fabricius and Aristotle in another sense too—by investigating and writing extensively in his manuscript notebooks on respiration, motion and generation. He may well have begun his research project with these areas chiefly in mind, and then branched off into other topics, in preparation for his discussions of the major organs and body parts during his lectures. At a certain point Harvey decided to focus on the heart.

Here again Harvey's intellectual guides were probably influential. According to Aristotle, the heart was the 'foundation of life', an all-important organ where blood was heated and became mingled with pneuma, the body's life-giving spirit or soul—an idea Galen had echoed. Fabricius may, instead, have inspired Harvey's decision because of his neglect of the heart. 'After having dealt carefully with almost all parts of animals', the Italian had, Harvey noted, 'left only the heart untouched'—the pupil could therefore complete his master's work. Harvey probably also concentrated on the heart because of the anomalies revealed by the preliminary investigations he made into the organ, perhaps in preparation for his lectures, his observations appearing inconsistent, in several respects, with traditional Galenic views. And then there was of course the heart's profound cultural significance, which prompted Harvey to examine an organ he regarded as the source 'of all affections', as the 'God' of the body and the citadel of the soul.

Over a series of evenings in the late 1610s and early 1620s Harvey attempted, through various 'trials' in his private research chamber, to finally settle the thorny questions he had touched on in his anatomical lecture on the heart, concerning the porous septum, the movement of the blood across the lungs, and the motion of the heart.

Harvey hauled the body of a hanged man on to his dissection table, doubtless with the help of a servant, anatomizing a cadaver being an enormous physical and practical challenge for one man. The corpse had been obtained through the auspices of the College of Physicians.

Having cut open the thorax and exposed the heart, Harvey tied (or ligated) the man's pulmonary artery. Introducing a tube through the vena cava to the right ventricle of the heart, he injected a large quantity of water into it with great force. The right ventricle swelled violently, until it seemed that it would burst. Yet 'not even a single drop', he observed, 'escaped through' the septum into the left ventricle. 'By my troth,' Harvey concluded, 'there are no pores, nor can they be demonstrated'—he was now certain that the all-powerful Galen had erred.

Releasing the ligature from the pulmonary artery Harvey then attempted to drive water into the lungs in order to test Colombo's notion of the pulmonary transit of the blood. After again injecting water into the vena cava, it almost instantly 'shot forward, mixed with a large amount of blood' out of the pulmonary artery and into the left ventricle. This convinced Harvey that blood passed 'from the right ventricle of the heart, into the lungs, and from thence into the left ventricle', via the pulmonary vein, just as Colombo had claimed.

Resolving the question of the movement of the heart—determining its active and passive phases—was a far more difficult proposition. The beating of the human heart could not be observed directly, but animals' hearts could be laid bare during vivisections. Colombo, whose Galenic focus was exclusively on human anatomy, had been forced to open up the thoraxes of living dogs, sheep and rabbits in his attempt to settle the issue; the Aristotelian Harvey regarded such experiments as routine.

Harvey now reprised Colombo's experiments in his private

chamber, cutting up animals night after night, week after week, year after year. Yet after these bloody trials the physician still found the matter murky, being unable to 'rightly perceive at first when the systole (contraction) and when the diastole (expansion) took place, by reason of the rapidity of the motion' of the animal's heart, which was 'accomplished in the twinkling of an eye, coming and going like a flash of lightning'.

Observation was slightly easier when an animal's 'heart began to die and move faintly, and life is as if it were departing'. The organ's motions then became 'slow and seldom, and the restings of longer continuance', as the heart 'yields, flags, weakens' and 'lyes as it were drooping'. The movements of the flagging heart seemed to bear out Colombo's idea that contraction was the active phase and expansion the passive. The motions were still not entirely clear to Harvey, however—nor indeed had they been to Colombo, whose account of the matter was at times ambiguous and obscure.

At some point in his investigations, Harvey's Aristotelian approach offered him a crucial inspiration. As his aim was to investigate the heart in *all* animals, he turned from hot-blooded to cold-blooded creatures. Toads, serpents, frogs, snails and all manner of little fishes now went under his knife. Colombo had never thought to examine these species, partly because he was not interested in the anatomy of the lesser animals per se, and partly because he studied organs in their broader physiological context rather than in Aristotelian isolation. Like Galen and Vesalius, Colombo investigated the heart as part of the respiratory system; this meant that fish, which do not have lungs, bore no relevance to his researches.

To his intense excitement, Harvey found that the hearts of cold-blooded animals beat far more slowly than those of warm-blooded creatures, so their movements were much easier to observe. Harvey held up to the artificial light of his private chamber a jar that contained 'a sort of very little fish, called in English a shrimp, taken in the River of the Thames'. Its body was transparent, 'the outward parts nothing at all obstructing' his sight, but acting 'like a window'. With the aid of a magnifying glass, its heart could be seen slowly expanding and contracting. Gazing intently at the shrimp, Harvey was convinced that he saw the blood leaving the heart 'through a pipe or artery', when the organ contracted.

To investigate further Harvey brought various containers full of fish over to his dissection table. Removing one of the larger creatures (a cod or barbell) he laid it down on the table and cut open its writhing body to expose its beating heart. He observed that, in a state of contraction, the fish's heart became smaller and narrower, as well as 'whiter in the tightening'. Putting his finger on the heart during systole, he noticed that it became 'relatively hard, like a muscle in contraction'. Harvey knew that 'all muscles in active movement gain in strength, contract, change from soft to hard, and thicken'; he felt this to be equally true of the fish's heart. Lengthy examination was impossible however, as the fish lay dead a short while after Harvey had cut it open, its tight white heart slowly turning into a flaccid chamber as it ceased to struggle.

Harvey also experimented on eels. Holding a wriggling eel down on the table, and tying its ends, he sliced it down the middle to reveal its heart. He then gouged the organ out with a blunt knife, as the heartless fish struggled violently and died. The bodiless heart continued to beat for a few seconds on the table; again, it seemed to become smaller, narrower and whiter in contracting. Harvey cut the organ up into little pieces and watched, enthralled, as the individual segments continued to beat to the same rhythm and in the same motion. What Harvey observed persuaded him that the heart was indeed a muscle whose active phase was contraction, not expansion as Galen had held. The Englishman was now sure that Colombo had guessed right, and he was equally sure that he could demonstrate this to others.

Buoyed up by his experiments on fish and eels, and having acquired from them what he believed to be a clearer understanding, Harvey returned, at some point, to his investigation of warm-blooded animals. He doubtless desired further confirmation of his conclusions; he also wished to investigate additional issues concerning the heart. Bringing a dog over to his dissection table, he tied it down, belly up, with the help of his servant. Exposing an animal's beating heart without killing it was a very delicate operation; if 'normal' living conditions were to be preserved for as long as possible the lungs must on no account be collapsed. Harvey's hands had to be steady and sure as he opened the thorax, bent back and broke the animal's ribs and cleared away the fat surrounding the heart.

Harvey gazed down at the dog's beating heart. What he saw appeared to confirm his idea of the blood's movement in and around the organ. Blood seemed to enter the right side of the heart via the vena cava. When the organ contracted, it appeared, he thought, to 'to drive out the blood as it were by force from the right ventricle, via the pulmonary artery into the lungs, and from thence to the left ventricle via the pulmonary vein', thus completing Colombo's 'pulmonary transit'. The contracting left ventricle, meanwhile, seemed to 'force blood into the aorta and so out into the rest of the body'.

To test this Harvey ligated the dog's vena cava. 'And here, wonderful to see, the pulmonary vein and pulmonary artery, along with the aorta' suddenly became 'empty of blood, and collapsed', their liquid supply cut off. The vena cava, on the other hand, was 'raised up with a great swelling; it beat on the obstructing barriers, vainly eager to break through'. Harvey then loosened the knots and 'suddenly the blood rushed into the empty chamber of the heart', and so through the pulmonary artery into the lungs.

Having established his conclusions regarding the blood's flow to his complete satisfaction, Harvey turned his attention to the arteries. These vessels appeared to dilate 'at the moment of contraction, impelled by the heart', rather than of their own accord, as Galen had suggested. The heart's contraction thus appeared to be the cause of the arterial pulse. Harvey tested this by ligating the aorta of the dog, which caused the pulse in that artery to cease, as well as an 'enlargement' and 'swelling' that 'almost ruptured' the left side of the heart. On releasing the knot, the flow of blood and the movement of the pulse in the aorta were immediately renewed. 'The pulse of the arteries', he concluded, 'was nothing but the impulsion of blood.'

At some point during his researches Harvey decided to slice through a dog's aorta at the moment of the heart's contraction, in a bid to investigate the amount and speed of the blood that was expelled by the heart in systole. Taking a knife, he cut down through the large artery. The blood immediately gushed out with force, and in copious quantity, in a series of expulsions. The spurts came intermittently, when the heart contracted, or so it seemed to Harvey. In a few seconds the tortured animal gave up the ghost, and the blood eventually stopped sputtering out of the perforated artery altogether. Here was another extraordinary anomaly. Most anatomists, following Galen, believed that the heart ejected only a very small amount of blood into the arteries, where it was supposed to gently ebb and flow in all directions, just as it did in the veins.

Many years later the goddess Fortune, or perhaps the gods of learning, rewarded Harvey for his patient labours by offering him the opportunity to examine a remarkable subject.

One day, the curious medical case of a young nobleman came to Charles I's ear. Apparently, as a child, the man had experienced a fall, which had caused a fracture in the ribs on the left side of his breast. A 'great quantity of putrified matter', as Harvey explained in his account of the incident, 'had been voided out of the wound', leaving the man with a wide gap open in his breast through which the movement of his lungs could, it was rumoured, be dimly perceived. His intellectual interest piqued, Charles dispatched Harvey to investigate.

Having explained to the young man the reason for his visit, Harvey 'opened the void part of his left side, taking off that small plate, which he wore to defend it against any outward injury'. There he beheld 'a vast hole in his breast, into which I could easily put my three Fore-fingers and my Thumb'. He soon perceived 'a certain fleshy part sticking out, which was driven in and out by a reciprocal motion, whereupon I gently handled it in my hand (without offense to the Gentleman)'. Amazed 'at the novelty of the thing' Harvey touched the fleshy substance repeatedly, and became convinced that it was not the lobe of the lungs, as most people supposed. Rather, what he was touching and gazing down at was 'the Heart and its Ventricles in their pulsation'. Harvey suddenly understood that he was realizing the dream dreamt by anatomists down the centuries, for neither Aristotle, Galen, Vesalius, Colombo nor Fabricius had ever seen or touched a beating human heart.

Harvey cleaned the wound then brought the young gentleman into the king's presence. During the ensuing examination Charles placed his hand in the young man's wound in order to touch his heart. His aim was to verify whether the heart, famed as the source of all feeling, was itself sensitive or deprived of sense. After testing the matter the king, along with his physician, concluded that the organ was incapable of feeling, 'For [the young man] perceived not that we touched him at all.'

Then Harvey invited his master to peer down closely into the wound, taking especial 'notice of the motion of the heart'— evidently *the* crucial issue for the physician. He asked the king to observe that 'the proper [i.e. active] motion of the heart is the Systole', when the blood is expelled from the organ; after careful examination Charles concurred with Harvey's conclusion.

And so the patient and lengthy observations Harvey had made on fish, toads and dogs had given him the clue to interpreting, and describing to witnesses, the movement of the heart of that most perfect animal, man.

❧ Essay 3 ❧

A short history of vivisection

FTER PUBLISHING ACCOUNTS of his private research in the two books he issued in the 1620s and 1650s, Harvey would become notorious, in the popular imagination, as the anatomist who 'arrived to a great proficiency in Cat and Dog cutting'. There were some, though, who admired his intrepidness in becoming one of the first English anatomists to cut up live animals, and probably the first dissector ever to turn his knife to cold-blooded creatures. Late seventeenth-century poets celebrated Harvey as a fearless explorer who 'plunged steel into the hearts / Of beasts, and gathered from the brutes' immortal knowledge.

An important part of Harvey's 'scientific' legacy is the sanction he gave to vivisecting animals. His innovative research suggested to some of his contemporaries, as well as to succeeding generations, that the practice bore rich fruit; his specific experiments on living animals were repeated throughout European universities later in the seventeenth century. To this day, Harvey remains the patron saint of pro-vivisectionists. Yet while Harvey was a pioneer so far as England was concerned, elsewhere the practice had a long history.

'Live cutting' was common in the ancient world, where animals were regarded as 'objects' without personalities or rights, which man (the master of creation) might use as he wished. Being bereft of rational souls and unable, in Aristotle's words, to 'learn all arts and workmanship, and handle an instrument with their hands', animals were believed to 'act not by art and intelligence but by natural instinct'. Yet for all of these differences, Aristotle and Galen held that direct parallels could be drawn between the *material* bodies of men and animals. Galen became famous in ancient Rome through his public vivisections on animals. The Greek physician was, however, so keen to emphasize the spiritual and intellectual distinction between animals and man that he rarely cut living apes, those 'imperfect, ridiculous, imitations of man'.

The vivisection (as well as the dissection) of humans was rumoured to have been carried out in Alexandria in the fourth century BC, the kings there apparently allowing anatomists to 'take criminals out of prison and dissect them alive, in order that they might probe the secrets of nature'. Virtually all natural philosophers and anatomists of the ancient world agreed, however, that the practice was abhorrent; Roman law forbade even the dissection of human corpses.

Christian theology adapted classical beliefs regarding animals. Man's rational soul was endowed with immortality; to argue that an animal had an immortal soul would be heresy. Animals, the medieval theologian St Thomas Aquinas declared, exist in a godless universe—the perpetual processes of feeding and copulation they participate in pertaining to the natural rather than the spiritual. They could not distinguish between true and false, or organize themselves into ordered and just societies—the hallmarks of rational beings. A promoter of the public dissection of human corpses for the greater glory of God, the Catholic Church also endorsed the vivisection of animals.

Vesalius described animal vivisections as 'the finishing touch to the whole course of anatomical study'; they also provided his courses with a suitably dramatic denouement. In the final dissection of one anatomy course he gave in Bologna, he 'took a dog, bound it with ropes to a small beam so that it could not move', but left it unmuz-zled. Above its terrified barking the Belgian tried to make himself heard: 'Now', he said, 'you will see in this living dog the function of the nervi reversivi [recurrent nerves].' He then opened the dog's thorax, located the two recurrent nerves around the arteries, and cut off one nerve. Half of the voice suddenly disappeared. Then he cut off the other nerve and the dog's bark could no longer be heard; 'only the breathing remained.' The students were suitably impressed, the 'mad' Italians among them becoming rowdy with excitement.

Colombo, a pupil of Vesalius, extended his master's explorations of the living animal body. The Italian described the vivisection of animals as necessary, medically useful and theologically and morally permissible. Colombo preferred to use dogs because bears and lions became too angry during vivisections, while pigs were 'too fat and noisy' for his liking. During the vivisection of a dog the Italian described the animal to his audience as 'happy' (i.e. lucky) 'because he affords to us a sight suitable for acquiring knowledge of the most beautiful things'.

Most of the great Renaissance anatomists prior to Harvey practised vivisection on animals. Philosophy and theology offered him countless reasons to justify his experiments. Common sense informed him that the practice was, in Francis Bacon's phrase, of 'great use' to the human race; it also suggested that if man killed animals in order to eat them, then doing so for the purposes of intellectual enlightenment must be a noble as well as a necessary endeavour.

Yet anatomists could not but feel pity for the creatures they tortured and killed on the dissection table, as well as guilt for doing so. The stoical Galen disliked cutting up living apes not only because they resembled men but also 'to avoid seeing their unpleasing expression when they were being vivisected'. Leonardo da Vinci recoiled in horror at the idea of inflicting pain on his 'fellow' creatures. Even the cold-hearted Colombo expressed sorrow, on occasion, for the 'poor dog', writhing beneath his knife. If only, one anatomist reflected, 'we could find a way to stupefy creatures' during vivisections, and thus render them insensible to the 'torture', then 'nobility' might be lent to the practice—but anaesthetics were three centuries away.

Jean Riolan the younger, anatomy professor at Paris University and perhaps the most celebrated European anatomist of the early seventeenth century, was the staunchest opponent of animal vivisection. He raised the spectre of two ancient fears surrounding the practice—that it would encourage the vivisection of humans, and that it would deaden the moral sensibility of both the anatomist and his audience. 'The anatomy of living animals', he warned, 'is similar to the slaughtering of living animals as it is performed by butchers. Encouraged through this kind of work, [butchers] do not hesitate to cut the throat of human beings for an unimportant reason. In the same way, anatomists who are accustomed to dissections of living animals will be ready to open secretly, moribund, but still living, human beings.' A number of voices joined Riolan to form a vocal anti-vivisection chorus, several anatomists among them even maintaining, in contradiction of the ancients, that the bodies of animals and men were too dissimilar for accurate comparisons to be made.

And so when Harvey bent over the bodies of animals in his research chamber, it is not the case, as has often been argued, that his culture had entirely desensitized him to the cruelty of his experiments. Certainly, if he wished to follow in the footsteps of Aristotle, Galen, Vesalius and Colombo, then it was almost inevitable that he would cut up living creatures; but pity, along with the arguments of Riolan, might have stayed his hand.

Unlike Colombo, Harvey is not known to have expressed any compunction whatsoever about inflicting the most appalling suffering on thousands of living animals. Perhaps concerned by this, his supporters felt the need to justify and excuse his vivisections. A Latin poem published soon after Harvey's death offers a fictional 'eyewitness' account of one of his experiments on a living dog. In the poem the animal's resistance to the vivisection, and its heart-rending distress, are vividly evoked. Flinching at the sight, the fictive Harvey explains to the few chosen friends comprising his audience that 'it is not ferocity of mind, nor dire lust that makes me cruel, nor the mercilessness of a wicked heart; but the sacred hunger for Fame', along with the desire to 'open the dark secrets of nature, to enquire the causes of things unknown'. Only these noble ends, he declares, could 'force me against my will to make such experiments, and drive away from my breast gentle feelings'.

Before wielding the knife, Harvey speaks to the dog itself. 'Thou, wretched one', he says apologetically, 'though thou wilt experience unspeakable pain, and wilt bear an unmerited punishment, thou shalt have in death a solace . . . for never will thy fame perish, and in the entire world thou wilt be renowned.' Harvey addresses the dog as a comprehending creature, and craves its pardon—an ostensibly 'modern' attitude that was in fact available to the seventeenth-century anatomist. But this is all fiction, and these are sentiments Harvey appears never to have uttered.

10. Birth of the theory (late 1610s–1620s): 'I began to bethink my self'

DURING HIS PRIVATE investigations Harvey had been impressed, and no doubt troubled, by the force and the amount of blood expelled by the contracting hearts of the various dogs whose aortas he severed. Conventional wisdom could not account for its quantity or intensity. According to tradition, blood was continually produced in the liver and consumed by the organs, muscles and tissues, reaching them after slow progress through the vessels. Yet if Harvey's observations regarding the large quantity of blood leaving the heart were correct, the liver would have to manufacture an inconcievably large amount of the liquid.

The vast amount of blood leaving the heart, along with its intensity, also seemed to lend credence to his idea that the organ's active phase was systole, a forceful contraction being required to evacuate the organ of so much liquid. Perhaps with an eye to convincing his fellow physicians and the audiences of his lectures on this latter point, Harvey set about trying to quantify the amount of blood leaving the heart and entering the arteries with every heartbeat. If he could come up with an impressively large figure, others might be persuaded of his views.

Harvey estimated the amount of blood present in the left

ventricle of the heart in passive diastole; then, deliberately keeping his calculations conservative, he speculated that only a fraction of that blood (roughly a drachm in weight) would be ejected at every systole. Harvey computed that in a single hour, during which the heart beat, at a low estimate, roughly 2,000 times, approximately 2,000 drachms would be expelled by the organ. This meant that over the course of one day, a little less than 50,000 drachms of blood would be ejected into the arteries.

Harvey simply could not believe that the liver was capable of producing so much blood; nor did he think it possible for men to consume the amount of food required (according to Galenic theory) to generate such an enormous quantity. Moreover, he could not understand either why the arteries did not swell, or even 'burst with too much intrusion of blood' from the contracting heart, or how the muscles, tissues and organs of the body could absorb it all. The body would surely become flooded with so much liquid, in the space of a few hours. Galen's 1,500-year-old theory began to appear incongruous or impossible.

Harvey then focused on the question of where all the blood went after it entered the aorta. Tradition taught him, and observation seemed to confirm, that the liquid was transported throughout the body via the arteries. To test this, Harvey devised a number of experiments on humans using ligatures, which he had often used during his medical practice when letting the blood of his patients.

Harvey tied a ligature as 'tightly as was bearable' just above the elbow of one of his servants, who was instructed to clasp a piece of wood in his hand. He noticed that 'beyond the ligature, towards the hand' no blood was able to flow through the arteries. He also saw that blood began to build up in the arteries above the ligature 'as if it were trying to burst through the passage and to reopen the channel.' Releasing the ligature just a little, Harvey observed an 'immediate coloration and distention of the whole hand.' It was evident that blood was carried to the extremities of the body by the arteries, and that its flow could be impeded.

But what of the veins? At a certain point Harvey decided to conduct some tests on these vessels too, no doubt taking inspiration from his old mentor Fabricius. Fabricius had conducted trials on the veins at Padua, possibly in front of Harvey and his fellow students. He gave an account of these in print, in his 1603 treatise *De venarum ostiolis* (*The little doors of the veins*), the 'little doors' being 'extremely delicate little membranes in the veins, occurring at intervals, singly or in pairs'.

The Italian investigated the function of 'little doors' by rubbing and squeezing, with his fingers, the distended veins in a man's ligated arm. Fabricius 'exerted pressure on the blood' in the veins in a bid to 'force it downwards' towards the hand. Yet he found that the liquid would not flow in that direction because it was, so far as he could see, 'held up and delayed' in the veins by the 'little doors'.

'My theory', the Italian concluded after these various trials, 'is that Nature has formed the little doors to delay the blood, and to prevent the whole mass of it flooding to the feet, or hands and fingers, and collecting there. The little doors are thus made to ensure a fair general distribution of the blood for the nutrition of the various parts.' This thesis made perfect sense within a Galenic view of the body in which the blood moved slowly around the vessels, in both directions, and needed to be sent out from the liver evenly and centrifugally to the various body parts.

Harvey repeated Fabricius' experiments in his private chamber. Ligating his servant's arm to swell the veins, he confirmed that blood was indeed prevented from flowing downwards in them by the 'little doors', no matter what pressure he exerted on it with his fingers. To test this further Harvey also ligated the exposed veins of vivisected animals, a little way above a pair of 'little doors'.

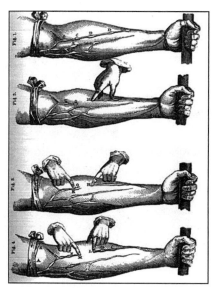

Figures from *De motu cordis*.

Despite the vast build-up of blood in the veins between the 'doors' and the ligature, the 'doors' would not allow blood to flow back downwards.

From these tests Harvey deduced something quite different from Fabricius. He hypothesized that the 'doors' must function like valves, encouraging the flow of blood in the veins in one direction, not simply delaying its movement as the Italian had thought. That direction was obviously not downwards but upwards—something confirmed by movement of the blood towards the shoulder when the pressure of the ligature was released in his servant's arm. Fabricius did not observe this unidirectional upward movement because his Galenic understanding of the blood within the body did not prompt him to look for it. Harvey, however, looked down at his servant's arm with a mind far more sceptical to Galen's theory.

At some point, Harvey had an inspiration which allowed him to look at the valves, and to consider their purpose, from an entirely original point of view. If they did not merely impede the downward flow of the blood 'from the large veins into the smaller ones, or from the centre of the body to the extremities' but actively facilitated its upward movement, then their central purpose might be to encourage the blood's passage 'from the extremities back to the centre'—that is, to the heart.

Harvey's understanding of the vast quantity and force of blood expelled by the contracting heart seems to have dovetailed in his mind with his attempt to map the blood's flow within the arteries and the veins. In endeavouring to resolve one issue—where all the blood went to—perhaps he might be able find the solution to the other.

> When [I] took notice that the valves in the veins . . . were so placed that they gave free passage of the blood towards the heart, but opposed the passage the other way: [I] was invited to imagine, that so provident a cause as nature had not plac'd so many valves without design: and no design seemed more probable, than that, since the blood could not well, because of the valves, be sent by the veins to the limbs, it should be sent [to the limbs] through the arteries [by the heart] and return [to the heart] through the veins . . . and when I had a long time considered with my self how great abundance of blood was passed through . . . I perceived that the veins should be quite emptied, and the arteries be burst with too much intrusion of blood, unless the blood did pass through arteries to the veins, and so return into the right ventricle of the heart.

The idea began to crystallize in Harvey's mind that, after the venous blood had been vivified in the lungs and conveyed to the left side of the heart, it was ejected by the contracting organ into the aorta, which distributed it throughout the body via the arteries. The blood was then transferred from the arteries to the veins—how and where Harvey could not say—before the veins conveyed the *same blood* back again to the vena cava at the right side of the heart in a closed system. The blood thus traced a double 'circuit'—one through the lungs, and one throughout the body. 'And so', Harvey recalled, 'I began to bethink my self if the blood might not have a circular motion . . .' This was the closest Harvey ever came to a 'eureka moment'.

✌ Essay 4 ✌

Francis Bacon, experiment, and empiricism

AN INDEFATIGABLE EXPERIMENTER, with a rare genius for devising and interpreting 'trials', it is hardly surprising that William Harvey has often been described as a practical counterpart of Francis Bacon (1561–1626), the great philosopher of empiricism. 'Bacon', one of Harvey's twentieth-century biographers wrote, 'laid down the rules for the collection of facts and for inductive methods of thought, but he did not sufficiently realize the value of experiment. Harvey by his example taught the correct place of experiment. The sequence was careful observation, thoughtful deliberation, appropriate experiment, and further consideration upon its results. This has ever since been the model for research students.'

Conveniently for those who make such claims, Bacon was one of Harvey's patients during the late 1610s and early 1620s. Harvey was rather wary of the super-subtle thinker and Machiavellian politician: Bacon's 'delicate, lively, hazel eie' reminded him of the 'eie of a viper'. It is likely that they clashed occasionally on medical matters. Bacon had his own ideas about how diseases ought to be treated, and rarely followed his doctor's orders.

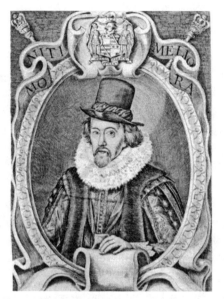

Portrait of Francis Bacon. Formerly King James I's Solicitor General, Attorney General and Lord Keeper, Bacon was elevated to Lord Chancellor in 1618 and given the title Baron Verulam.

Bacon was sorely afflicted with gout throughout his adult life: 'never beggar', he would wail like a titan in pain, 'had the gowte but me'. He probably called on Harvey during one of his many attacks. A veteran of the malady himself, Harvey was certainly qualified to suggest a number of treatments. 'If you would be rid of the gout', the physician told his patients, 'you must neither drinck wine nor any strong drinck; you must eate but once a day, and that sparingly too.' Bacon probably demurred, as he believed that a combination of plasters, poultices and baths would see off an attack. It seems unlikely, though, that his proud physician would have obliged him by carrying out the proposed treatment.

Bacon had a low opinion of physicians generally, dismissing most of them as charlatans. In his famous treatise on education *The*

Advancement of Learning (1605), he argued that medicine had progressed little, if at all, in the modern period. It relied too heavily on authorities, when inductive investigation was required. 'Men have withdrawn themselves too much from the contemplation of nature, and the observations of experience, and have tumbled up and down in their own reason and conceit . . . they [have been] made fierce with dark keeping.' Bacon proposed a new philosophic system, based on the empirical examination of nature. 'All depends on keeping the eye steadily fixed on the facts of nature, and so receiving their images simply as they are.'

'My way of discovering sciences [i.e. knowledge]', Bacon wrote, 'performs everything by the surest rules.' These rules included the compilation of detailed statistical tables relating to all the manifestations and variations of a particular phenomenon—for example, that of heat. Surveying the mass of particular instances garnered in these tables, Bacon believed that he was in a position to isolate what was essential about a phenomenon. By a process of induction, he could, he argued, also arrive at general hypotheses regarding it. These hypotheses could in turn be tested by experiments 'skilfully and artificially devised for the express purpose of determining the point in question'.

Bacon criticized thinkers such as Plato for 'intermingling' '[natural] philosophy with theology', yet the main target of his prose polemics was Aristotle. The Greek philosopher's 'four causes' of natural phenomena should, he argued, be dispensed with, especially the final cause which confounded men's minds by focusing on the ultimate purpose or the 'why' of phenomena. This was something that, in his view, simply could not be fathomed—nor did it need to be.

Bacon claimed that Aristotelian syllogisms were flawed too, being based on 'propositions which consisted of words'—that is the 'symbols of notions'. The problem was that 'if the notions themselves are confused there can be no firmness'. Moreover, syllogisms encouraged men to argue from a universal principle (i.e. 'All men are mortal') to a particular (i.e. 'Socrates is a man'), when what they ought to be doing was using particular instances as stepping stones towards general principles. Aristotle was, Bacon complained, liable to entangle men's minds in a net of words and propositions; this rendered them pedantic and sluggish when it came to identifying facts. The Greek's philosophy was an inadequate tool for 'enquiring into truth', utterly 'useless for the discovery of knowledge'.

Bacon saw some promise in the innovative ideas and methods of contemporary natural philosophers such as Galileo, who had been Padua University's professor of mathematics during Harvey's time there. Like Bacon, Galileo believed that natural philosophy ought to be based on 'sensory experience and necessary demonstration' rather than an abstract exploration of the 'why' of things. Bacon admired Galileo's experiments to establish the precise measurement of the primary qualities of external bodies—their size, shape, quantity and motion—the Italian maintaining that these were the only qualities inherent in objects; secondary qualities, such as colour or scent, existed partly in men's minds.

Yet even the great Tuscan was found wanting by Bacon, for the limited scope and number of his experiments. He complained that Galileo's 'trials' stopped 'with [a] few discoveries'—that is, after his tests had settled a theory to his satisfaction—'and [so] many other things equally worthy of investigation are not discovered by the same means'. Galileo still dedicated too much time to imaginative philosophical thought for the English empiricist. 'Individual excellence' or 'genius' was, Bacon held, far less important than the establishment of a broad, state-funded programme of experimentation into all natural phenomena, carried out by humble artisans who would use their eyes and hands as much as their minds. The knowledge accrued from such a project would, Bacon prophesied, give man dominion over the entire natural world, as well as the power to harness its energies and resources.

Bacon believed that technological advances such as printing, gunpowder and the compass had already 'changed the whole face and state of things throughout the world'; the exploration of distant lands beyond Europe had also revealed new wonders. And there were still so many secrets to uncover, myriad domains to map and master, numerous instruments to devise, countless natural forces to manipulate and exploit. Through induction and empirical investigation man would be restored to the pristine condition of perfection and potency he had enjoyed before the Fall; in action he would be like an angel, in apprehension, like a God!

Over the course of his private research, Harvey tested various hypotheses, such as the forceful systole, by devising experiments on human cadavers and living animals, and observing the results. His 'trials' revealed a number of anomalies in traditional notions of the function of the heart and the movement of the blood, and he appears to have formulated alternative theories that were in better keeping with his findings.

At first glance, Harvey's project would appear to have been thoroughly Baconian, as does his achievement in undermining a 1,500-year-old theory through empirical investigation and the discovery of anomalous facts. Harvey overpowered tradition, it seems, because he was an empiricist, no longer content to rely on books, but determined instead to investigate the body *as it really is*. When discussing his methodology, Harvey always emphasized the importance of ocular testimony, the reading of books being less important than 'finding out the nature of things by the things themselves'. Harvey's innovative circulation theory, it has often been argued, emerged organically from a revolutionary Baconian method.

Harvey's methods and philosophy were, however, utterly different from Bacon's. The empirical aspect of his research programme, like most of its other facets, was derived from Aristotle, the 'general' whose authority carried such weight with the Englishman that he 'never did think of differing from him inconsiderately'.

It may have been at Padua that Harvey had learned of Aristotle's theories regarding the role of particulars, and empirical enquiry, in the search for universal philosophical knowledge. These theories were far more subtle than Bacon's polemics suggested. 'Singulars are to us more known', the Greek philosopher wrote, 'and are the first to exist according to the information of sense, for there is nothing in the understanding which was not first in the sense . . . and we more readily define singulars than universals, for there is more equivocation in universals; whence it is advisable to pass from singulars to universals . . . It is impossible to have universal theoretical propositions without induction.' Harvey quoted this passage in his published writings, as a statement of his personal philosophic faith. He also cited in print Aristotle's famous suggestion that: 'If one day things become sufficiently known, then will the evidence of the senses be more worthy to be believed than reason. Reason, indeed is only to be believed when those things which are demonstrable in argument agree with those things which are perceived by the senses.'

Harvey's 'general' had advocated a continual interchange between individual facts and general theories, observation and reason, particular instances and universals, as the basis of true natural philosophy. An Aristotelian had no interest in facts divorced from a broader philosophic context—to establish the dimensions or weight of an object by quantitative experiments, for instance, was meaningless in itself.

Harvey's most famous experiment was his measurement of the quantity of the blood leaving the heart at the moment of contraction. In testing this, it has often been suggested that he proceeded along Baconian lines. After close observation, he devised the hypothesis that blood leaves the heart, in systole, in a considerable quantity. The next step was to establish how much blood was ejected with every contraction.

Yet Harvey was not interested in the exact amount of the blood ejected by the heart as an isolated fact—the fact was, in itself, of little use to him. What he wanted to demonstrate was that a *great deal* of blood left the heart, in order to illustrate just how forceful the systole was, and to suggest that more blood was ejected than could either be accommodated comfortably by the arteries or produced by the liver.

Accordingly, Harvey made an extremely rough estimate of the amount of blood leaving the contracting heart, based on the volume of blood contained in the left ventricle. Had he wanted to be more exact, he could have measured the amount of blood spurting out of a perforated aorta (and then multiplied it by the number of heartbeats per minute). In his lifetime, other anatomists would devise the means to make this very measurement, but even when their procedure was well known, Harvey did not adopt it to arrive at a more accurate figure. He neglected to carry out this test because exactitude was not his aim; what he required was a convincing illustration for his theory, as it were, for rhetorical effect. Neither Bacon, nor Galileo, who performed precise quantitative experiments, would have proceeded in this fashion.

There were, as a matter of fact, fundamental philosophical differences between Harvey and Galileo. Harvey always denied the Italian's crucial distinction between the primary qualities of an external body, which could be quantified, and its secondary qualities, which could not. When Harvey came to make 'ocular inspection' of an animal or human body, he was as interested in its secondary as he was in its primary qualities, citing both as equally weighty 'evidence' for his theories. It may be worth remarking here on Harvey's apparent lack of interest in attending any of Galileo's lectures during his stay at Padua; he seems never to have sought out the professor of mathematics or to have troubled himself about the Italian's ideas.

Unlike Bacon (and to a much greater extent than Galileo) theory invariably informed and preceded observation for Harvey, the universal truth coming before the individual fact. Aristotle's deductive principles, rather than empirical data, were the starting point for his enquiries. In his investigations into the movement of animal muscles, for example, Harvey began with the following Aristotelian first principles: 'Nature is the principle of motion and change'; 'Nature in the making of muscles is concerned with two things, their actions and functions'; 'Nature does nothing that can be done by fewer', and 'The soul working within the body is the basis and pattern for all movement'. He then proceeded to examine how these principles were embodied in particular animals.

Aristotelian first principles were also present in his mind throughout his investigations into the heart. When Harvey observed 'the symetrie, and magnitude of the ventricles of the heart and of the vessels which go into it', and especially the 'carefull artifice' of the valves, he reflected that, '*since nature does nothing in vain*', and since 'so provident a cause as nature' could not have 'plac'd so many valves without design', the vessels and the valves *must* have a *purpose*—which, ultimately, had to be the circulation of the blood. Harvey was expressing the Aristotelian belief that the organs of the body were all designed with an end in mind, and that nature had an aim or 'final cause' bestowed upon it by God—a truth that Bacon's philosophy denied.

Harvey claimed that his theory had been 'confirmed by many ocular demonstrations' and 'illuminated by reasons and arguments'. It was this Aristotelian interplay between data and ideas, between magnificent generalizations and particulars, that prompted Harvey's theory. Facts, to adapt his own metaphor, were the labyrinth; ideas and Aristotelian principles, his Ariadne's thread.

Bacon's writings were greatly admired by the courtiers and scholars of England. In both private conversation and in print Harvey complimented Bacon for 'for his wit and style', his prose being among the very finest. Yet, much to the chagrin of those modern commentators who depict the pair as intellectual allies, Harvey 'would not', according to a friend, 'allow [Bacon] to be a great philosopher'. 'He writes Philosophy', Harvey would say in a tone of derision, 'like a Lord Chancellor—I have cured him.' As the Lord Chancellor presided over the legal courts, Harvey may have been implying that Bacon wrote like a barrister, who regards truth as something to be proven by factual evidence rather than philosophical ingenuity, and who is motivated by the goal of practical social utility, instead of that of attaining true knowledge.

In quipping that he had 'cured' his patient, Harvey could have been alluding to an intellectual joust between the pair at which Bacon was worsted, or perhaps the phrase expresses the doctor's belief that his life's work offered a philosophical riposte to Bacon's manifestos of empiricism and his attacks on Aristotle. 'To [think you can] go beyond Aristotle', Bacon had written, using 'the light of Aristotle' is to 'think that a borrowed light can increase the original light from which it is taken'. Harvey's research into the heart and the blood would disprove that elegant epigram.

One thing is certain: by announcing that he had 'cured' Bacon, Harvey was not referring to having eradicated his lordship's gout, which only became more 'ambitious' with time, changing its 'old course', by migrating from toe to heel.

11. Demonstration (late 1610s–1620s): 'Whereby I offer you to perceive and judge'

HARVEY WORKED AWAY in his private research chamber, experimenting, observing, making inferences and connections; yet he was not alone there. A number of figures can be glimpsed among the shadows around his dissection table, various gentlemen who (as one of the group put it) 'scrutinized' every movement of Harvey's hand with 'sharp and lynx-like eyes', and weighed his every word.

Having developed his circulation theory and established it to his own satisfaction with various 'trials', Harvey now 'showed' it to other people, in an attempt to persuade them of his opinion. The showing of Harvey's theory would take place over countless sessions, during a period of about ten years (roughly between 1618 and 1628), in which Harvey's private chamber was transformed into a public theatre. Harvey may also have demonstrated certain aspects of his theory during his Lumleian lectures at Amen Corner.

Opinions in natural philosophy had to be shown to 'reliable' witnesses, who might then vouch for them, thus altering their status from proposed hypotheses to truths and facts. The philosophical status of factual truths was a matter of controversy; their empirical validity was also often called into question. Only certain groups, with approved social and intellectual status, had the power to establish them. In accounts of his experiments, Harvey would invariably emphasize the civil as well as the scholarly standing of his witnesses, informing readers that he often demonstrated his theories to the king himself.

The men who crowded around Harvey's dissection table, were, in his words, the 'clear-sighted folk' and 'most learned men' who comprised the College of Physicians. The best view of the proceedings was reserved for Dr John Argent, the college's president, a man Harvey called his 'singular friend'. Throughout the discourse that accompanied his demonstrations, Harvey invoked the testimony and approval of Argent, which carried a great deal of weight with the other witnesses, by frequently prefacing his descriptions of observations with: 'I have seen—as Dr Argent will be my witness . . .'.

Harvey announced that he would propose an entirely new opinion concerning the motion and use of the heart and the movement of the blood. 'I will affirm', he declared to his no doubt wonder-wounded hearers, 'my most excellent Doctors, the blood to pass forth and return through unwonted tracts, contrary to the received way, through so many ages of years insisted upon, and evidenced innumerable, and by the most famous and learned men.'

Probably speaking for the most part in Latin, Harvey offered his theory as a proposal for the consideration of his learned audience— '*quare vobis cernendum et judicandum proponum*' ('whereby I offer you to perceive and judge').

I affirm that the blood does first pass through the lungs into the left ventricle, and is forcibly ejected from the contracting left ventricle to all parts of the body via the arteries, and does creep into the veins and porosities of the flesh, stealing into the remotest corners of the body to nourish them. From there it returns from the little veins into the greater, comes at last into the vena cava, in so great abundance, with so great flux and reflux, so that it cannot be furnished by those things which we do take in, and in a far greater abundance than is competent for nourishment. It must be of necessity concluded that the blood is driven with force and speed in a circular motion, and that it moves perpetually; and hence does arise the action and function of the heart, which by pulsation causes this motion.

Harvey explained that he would confirm the theory by various ocular demonstrations; he urged his audience to evaluate these trials not so much with their knowledge of anatomical tradition, as with their senses—that is, to '*see for themselves*'. His demonstrations would be accompanied by reasons and arguments. When his presentation had been concluded, the audience would be at liberty to raise any objections that had occurred to them, which Harvey would then endeavour to address. In other words, the presentation would proceed in an academic fashion, in the formal style of a university dispute, the theory being stated, demonstrated and supported with argument, before being challenged and defended. Only if it withstood this rigorous scholastic test would the thesis be considered valid.

Over numerous sessions, Harvey showed his colleagues the various facets of this theory: the impervious septum, the pulmonary transit, the forceful systole, the function of the valves, the quantity and force of the blood leaving the heart with every beat and the movement of the blood within the arteries and the veins. In the process, he cut up countless cadavers and living animals, and supported his inferences with elaborate philosophical arguments.

The fellows of the college then attacked his theories with all the ardour of undergraduates. Numerous specific criticisms were aired. Certainly, one observed, a great deal of blood spurted out from the perforated veins and arteries around the heart of a living animal, but exactly how much blood leapt forward, and might not the amount be explained by the unnatural violence Harvey was doing to the animal's heart? Could, another asked, a noble organ such as man's heart really be investigated by exploring the body of an eel—surely the bodies of fish and men were too dissimilar to draw comparisons? And then there was the thorny issue of the forceful systole, the ocular demonstration of which was inconclusive even to the most acute pair of eyes in the audience. Harvey's interpretation was not susceptible to demonstration, it was objected; furthermore it directly challenged the ideas of Galen.

The intellectual authority of the men who stood around Harvey's dissection table was inextricably associated with that of the Greek physician. Any fellow of the college practising treatments that contradicted Galenic theory was formally reprimanded; the college statutes forbade all criticism of the Greek. And yet here was 'honest' William Harvey—who had sworn to comply with those statutes and to promote the power of the institution—openly attacking its intellectual patron.

Nor was Harvey criticizing the 'all-powerful Galen' on specific points only. If true, his circulation theory would completely overthrow the Greek's concept of the function of the heart and the movement of the blood. Galen had held that there were two different types of blood and two almost entirely distinct vascular systems; Harvey was now proposing one of each. Where Galen's two systems were open, with most of the blood consumed by the muscles, tissues and organs and replaced continually in the liver, Harvey was suggesting a closed system with *the same blood* flowing perpetually around the body. And while Galen had argued that the blood's movement within the vessels was in various directions, in a slow ebb and flow rather like the tides of the sea, Harvey claimed the blood coursed rapidly through the veins and arteries like a gushing river and in one direction only.

And if Harvey's heart replaced Galen's, then the Greek's general vision of the internal workings of the body would have to be dispensed with. For Galen, man's organs functioned autonomously, actively drawing to themselves whatever substances, such as blood, they required for nourishment. If, however, the blood's flow around the body was caused and regulated by the contraction of the heart, then the role of the organs was diminished to that of passive receptacles. Moreover, the liver, paramount in Galen's system by virtue of the fact that it produced blood, was now relegated to a minor position within the body's hierarchy, the heart becoming the principal organ.

For Galen, the four humours remained largely separate within the body, and tended to dwell in specific areas; yet if blood coursed around the body, quickly and in copious quantities, then the humours would become mingled in a confused cocktail. The heart was supposed to regulate the harmonious distribution of the humours, not mix them up. The confusion of the humours was, Galenists believed, a major cause of sickness; Harvey's theory seemed to suggest it was the body's normal and healthy state.

There were times when the debate in Harvey's chamber became fractious, with some of the fellows offering barbed criticisms of Harvey, whose theory was undoubtedly construed as an attack on the Galenic medical therapies they employed daily. Bloodletting, for example, was applied to a specific afflicted area of the body in order to rebalance the humours there; the treatment would make no sense at all if the humours were promiscuously commingled within the body, or if the blood moved continually and quickly around it. Harvey's colleagues staunchly defended such practices, declaring that they had been efficacious in countless cases down the centuries. Not only did Galenic therapies work, but they also *had* to work, if the physicians' right to demand huge fees was to continue.

Harvey anticipated hostility from his colleagues on such points. It was only fitting, he realized, that physicians endeavour 'to keep Galen's medicine in good order'. He knew too that they would judge his new theory largely by the contribution it made to medical therapies, rather than from a philosophical or anatomical standpoint. He endeavoured to allay their fears by saying: 'I do not believe that my theory destroys Galenic medicine; rather it enhances it.' As an example, Harvey claimed that it explained why medicine taken into the mouth should produce beneficial effects all around the body—the circulating blood conveying the remedy quickly to all corners of the microcosm. It was a compelling argument, but one that offered cold comfort to his audience, many of whose favoured therapies would be rendered obsolete. On the specific issue of bloodletting, Harvey strove to appease his opponents, admitting that 'daily experience satisfies us that it has a most salutary effect in many diseases', whatever his new theory might suggest to the contrary. Harvey was clearly in earnest, but the contradictory nature of his position left him vulnerable to attack.

Harvey spent much of the debate on the defensive. He attempted to disarm his opponents with the assurance that it would not be a 'base' or 'shamefull' thing for them 'to change their opinions' or 'to desert their errors', however ancient those erroneous opinions might be. 'For true philosophers', he said, 'do not suffer themselves to be addicted to the slavery of any man's precepts; nor do they swear Allegiance to Mistris Antiquity, so openly to leave their friend Truth.'* As a variation on this theme he appealed to their sense of history. 'You are not so narrow spirited,' he told them, 'to believe that an art or science is so absolutely and perfectly taught in all points, that there is nothing remaining to the diligence and industry' of modern men.

Harvey's attempts to deflect criticism were largely ineffective, and the onslaught of objections continued. The anatomist may have been forced to present his theory as an abstract philosophical exercise, rather than as a contribution to practical medical theory.

---

* Here Harvey unconsciously echoes Leonardo da Vinci, who wrote: 'I will quote something far greater than [scholarly authority]: experience, the mistress of all [the scholars'] masters.' Leonardo's biographer, Charles Nicholl, discerns a 'touch of social defiance' in these words, as though 'his underprivileged beginning as an illegitimate son in a rural backwater . . . is being turned into a strength'. We can hear the same note in some of Harvey's pronouncements; his lowly origins undoubtedly informed the independence, originality and tenacity of his intellectual vision.

At times, the strain of the argument proved too much for him; at one point, he lost his temper, accusing his detractors of opposing him out of 'indignation and envy'.

And yet, in 1628, after almost a decade of argument and demonstration, Harvey felt confident enough to finally declare himself victor of the disputation. 'I have', he wrote to the fellows of the college, 'propounded [my theory] to you, confirmed it by ocular testimony, [and] answered your doubts and objections' so successfully and completely, as to have received 'the President's verdict in my favour'.

It is impossible to believe, however, that Harvey fully overcame his intransigent colleagues; it is indeed almost certain that Harvey's 'particular friend' Dr Argent reached a judgement in his 'favour' *despite* the fact that Harvey had failed to convince all, or even the majority, of his audience. Argent may have been persuaded by Harvey's demonstrations and arguments. He may also have trusted the conservative Harvey to keep the college's best interests at heart. Harvey was, after all, one of the rising stars of the institution, both in intellectual terms, and also socially, given his close association with the king. Argent may even have been grooming him as a future president.*

Now that he could call on the College ('being worthy of credit') as witness, Harvey dared to hope that a book elucidating his theory would 'come abroad entire and safe'—that is, be well received by the scholarly community. Without the imprimatur of an institution

---

* Argent's successors would not look so favourably on the circulation theory. Perhaps in consequence of the embarrassment that the publication of Harvey's theory would cause them, the college issued a new decree enabling the president and the fellows to censor all books written by fellows. As we shall see, several members of the order wrote direct and hostile attacks on the theory, which the college neglected to veto; the college also refused to publicly endorse the writings of fellows who rallied to Harvey's defence. For decades after the publication of Harvey's theory, lecturers at Amen Corner would either ignore, or contradict it during their anatomical demonstrations.

made 'famous by so great men', publication of his theory might have seemed 'an action too full of arrogancy'; having received Argent's blessing, Harvey was ready to prepare a treatise for the press.

He began writing in the mid to late 1620s, probably in one of the leather-bound folio manuscript notebooks he generally used for his compositions. Harvey scribbled fast in black ink on the right-hand page only. His hand was spidery and uneven—a characteristic believed to be common in learned men. It was said by a friend that 'scarce any man' could read his ostentatiously 'obscure' manuscripts without difficulty. Yet legibility may not have been essential at this stage as Harvey is likely to have begun with a rough working draft.

As Harvey jotted down his thoughts, words elided, lines were linked, certain letters became indistinguishable. The letters 'u' and 'a' were almost identical, as were 'e' and 'o'. The letters 'm' and 'n' were often omitted from the middle or end of a word. He generally abbreviated words, and was eccentric, even by the erratic standards of the time, in his punctuation, capitalization and spelling. Harvey generally crossed out and revised as he went, squeezing in alternative words above and below his original text. He scrawled in the margins, both vertically and horizontally, in the process covering every inch of the recto. More substantial second thoughts, and longer additions, were written on the verso page, opposite the relevant section of text. For particularly lengthy interpolations, he usually wrote on a separate single manuscript sheet, which he then inserted into the notebook between the appropriate pages. As was his custom when structuring an argument, Harvey generally annotated his text with 'X', 'WH' and symbols such as 'Δ'—the latter representing something that had been demonstrated.

The Latin which flowed from Harvey's quill was often as rugged as the hand in which it was written. 'Good God!' reads the English translation of one of his favourite exclamations; 'By my troth!' was another. With his homely, vivid style Harvey transported the reader to his research chamber, setting him down right beside the dissection table. 'Upon a time', he wrote, 'trying an experiment upon a [vivisected] Dove, after that the heart had quite left motion, and that the ears [of the heart] had quite given over, I wetted my finger with spittle, and being warmed kept it a while upon the heart; by this fomentation, as if it had received strength and life afresh, the heart and its ears began to move, to contract, and open, and did seem as it were recall'd back again from death.'

In plain, vigorous prose, the country boy from Kent depicted nature as he saw it—in infinitesimal detail. He had a genius too for illuminating the unfamiliar interior of the body with everyday metaphors: 'the arteries are stretched', he remarked of the entrance of the blood into these vessels, 'because they are fill'd like Baggs or Satchels' or 'as your gloves would if you blew into them, increasing in volume in all of its fingers'. Striking similes followed lucid arguments and evocative vignettes as the manuscript grew under Harvey's hand.

✑ Essay 5 ✑

The landscape of Harvey's imagination (I):
Microcosm and macrocosm

ARVEY SET ASIDE a special 'meditating apartment' in his London home, and in the grounds of a country house he purchased at Combe he had some caves dug 'in the Earth, in which in Summer time he delighted to meditate'. Believing darkness and quiet to be 'best' for 'contemplation', Harvey relished the calm of these retreats. The work of 'trial' and observation suspended, he would sit still for hours at a time, reflecting on his studies in sanctuaries that were the very antithesis of his noisy, gory, candlelit research chamber.

The thinking Harvey did in his meditating apartment was undoubtedly as significant for his treatise as the investigations he conducted in his research chamber. Today, we tend to emphasize the importance of the latter because the laboratory has, over the last century, become the only arena in which 'truth' can be faithfully tested. Moreover, many people now regard the brain as a mere *camera obscura* on to which a 'true' image of reality is mechanically projected via our eyes. That is why, in numerous modern accounts, Harvey is praised not for the subtlety of his thought, but for the clearness of his vision: putting theory and tradition (those 'chimeras' of the mind) to one side, he saw what others could not see—the truth of nature.

Yet Harvey's brain was no passive receptacle, but rather an active, vital, creative agent, with distinct contours and modes of classification and association. These were inevitably informed by intellectual theories and beliefs common to the general and scholarly culture of the seventeenth century, and influenced by the conventional phrases and metaphors of the time. Such cultural elements had animated and directed Harvey's research from the very beginning; now, as he wrote his treatise, they would condition his analysis and his theories.

None of this should surprise us. A natural philosopher can no more stand outside of his intellectual and cultural horizon than a poet, a social commentator, or a preacher; like them, he must express himself, and think, in the concepts and language of his period. Harvey's contemporaries appreciated this—according to popular opinion only Adam had been able to see the world *as it really is*, but he had forfeited this blessed vision by his disobedience in the Garden of Eden. If we are, therefore, to understand the treatise that Harvey was now penning, it must be read alongside the productions of contemporary writers working in other genres and disciplines. Their work, along with the treatise itself, allows us to peer into, and to illuminate, the dark meditating chamber that was Harvey's mind.

'The heart', Harvey wrote in his treatise, 'is a Prince [i.e. a king] in the Commonwealth, in whose person is the first and highest government every where.'* The anatomist was drawing upon the

---

*The quotations which appear here, and in the following two essays, are mostly taken from the first English translation of *De motu cordis*, which was published in 1653, a quarter of a century after the Latin original was issued in 1628. I have also quoted some of Harvey's near contemporary unpublished writings (such as his lecture notes), in order to illustrate general points concerning his style, method of composition, or his understanding of the heart and the blood.

common idea of the body politic—the notion that society can be likened to the human body, and vice versa. 'As it hath pleased God', a contemporary social commentator wrote, 'to make the body of divers parts and members, and every part and member hath his distinct and proper office . . . so hath it pleased God to ordain in the common-wealth divers degrees of people.' Yeomen were likened to the 'liver-veins of the Commonwealth' because they 'yielded good juice and nourishment to all other parts thereof'.

When Harvey looked down at a human corpse, he saw the body politic as well as the body anatomical. 'Nature performs her works in animals [including man]', he wrote, 'and attains her end by means of rhythm and harmony [in the muscles] . . . And thus it is too with the human good in the State, nothing is more excellent than the union of citizens in friendship, nothing better than order, and the virtue of the citizen is to continue in orderliness, and of the governor to be steadfast in duty and order.' At some level of thought no longer accessible to us today, for Harvey and his contemporaries the body was not simply *like* society, or society *like* the body; the body actually *was* society and vice versa. This notion is enshrined in a sixteenth-century judgement concerning the legal definition of the monarch: it was declared that 'The King has *in him* two Bodies: a Body natural, [which is] a Body mortal, and a Body politic, consisting of Policy and Government.'

The body politic was informed by an organic, God-ordained and profoundly conservative vision of society. It emphasized the importance of order, the preservation of the status quo through the restriction of social mobility, and the need to balance various, potentially conflicting, forces. 'Who did ever see', one clergyman asked, 'the feet and legs divide themselves from the head and other superior parts?' The monarch was vital to the healthy functioning of the body politic: he maintained harmony by regulating the humours of the social body, purging 'the proud, cholerick and melancholick' substances whenever required by decisive localized intervention. It was in this context that the king's 'sacred hands' were believed to be 'sweetn'd with that sacred salutiferous gift of Healing which supports the Body Politick and keeps up the Denizens and Subjects thereof in vigor and courage', the monarch thereby having the power to miraculously cure scrofula (the 'Kinges-Evill') through the laying on of hands.

John Donne (1572–1631), the poet of sensual and religious ecstasy, and dean of St Paul's Cathedral, scattered references to the body politic throughout his writings.

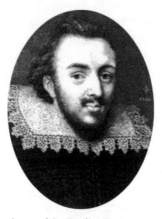

Portrait of Donne. As dean of St Paul's, Donne conducted a great deal of business with the College of Physicians over land and property; the fellows often attended Donne's services.

Well versed in the 'grounds and use of physick', and curious enough about anatomy to read Colombo, and perhaps even to attend Harvey's lectures, Donne's work is full of anatomical allusions, some of which concern the function and structure of the human heart. In the poem 'Of the Progresse of the Soule' he asks his reader:

> Know'st thou how blood, which to the heart doth flow,
> Doth from one ventricle to th' other goe?

In a sermon preached before King James, whose Royal Chaplain Donne was from 1615 to 1621, he returned to the organ: 'We know the receipt', he declared, 'the capacity of the ventricle . . . of all the receptacles of the blood, how much blood the body can have . . . When I look into the larders, and cellars, and vaults, into the vessels of our body for drink, for blood, for urine, they are pottles and gallons.'

More often, however, Donne places the human heart in the context of the body politic. In one of his devotional writings he hailed James I as the 'heart' of the Commonwealth. 'Since the heart hath the birthright and Primogeniture . . . the first part which is first borne . . . the Heart alone is in the Principalitie, and in the Throne, as King, the rest as subjects . . . [who] must contribute to that, as Children to their parents . . . this contribution of assistance of all to the Soveriegne, of all parts to the Heart, is from the very dictates of Nature.'

The King would have enjoyed his chaplain's recondite musings. James I was a vociferous defender of the divine right of kings, believing that the monarch was not subject to any earthly authority, parliamentary or religious, having been anointed by God; he also held it his subjects' duty to subsidize his court through their taxes.

For the dedication placed at the head of his treatise, Harvey composed a strikingly similar anatomical hymn of praise for James' son Charles, an equally vocal spokesman for the theory of the divine right, and a king whose rule was widely criticized as absolutist. Harvey offered his treatise to his royal master 'the Most Illustrious and Invincible Monarch / Charles / King of Great Britain, France, and Ireland, / Defender of the Faith'; 'Most Gracious King!' the dedication read:

> The Heart of creatures is the foundation of life, the Prince of all, the Sun of their Microcosm, on which all vegetation does depend, from whence all vigour and strength does flow. Likewise the King is the foundation of his Kingdoms, and the Sun of his Microcosm,

the Heart of his Commonwealth, from whence all power and mercy proceeds. I was so bold to offer to your Majesty those things which are written concerning the Heart, so much the rather, because all things human are according to the pattern of man, and most things in a King according to that of the Heart; Therefore the knowledge of his own Heart cannot be unprofitable to a King, as being a divine resemblance of his actions. You may at least, best of Kings, being plac'd in the top of human things, at the same time contemplate the Principle of Man's Body, and the Image of your Kingly power. I therefore must humbly intreat, most gracious King, accept, these new things concerning the Heart, [you] who are the new light of this age, and indeed the whole Heart of it, a Prince abounding in vertue and grace, to whom we acknowledge our thanks are due, for any good that England receives.

Harvey was an ardent monarchist devoted to his king, in the steadfast manner typical of yeomen who 'having once seen the King, pray for him every night thereafter'. Harvey threw his intellectual weight behind his monarch whenever possible, publicly upholding his exclusive claim to the divine inspiration by which he cured his subjects of the 'Kinges-Evill', inserting monarchical references into his demonstrations whenever he could. In a discourse on digestion, during one of his lectures, Harvey compared the acid rising up from the stomach to a motion sent from the Lower to the Upper House in Parliament, which suggests the low esteem in which he, and other monarchists, held that institution.

Harvey was not simply dressing up his treatise as monarchical propaganda, in the hope of receiving Charles I's patronage, blessing, and imprimatur. He was rehearsing his deeply held belief that the heart was as important for the body politic as the king was for the commonwealth and that the organ and monarch functioned in the same way and corresponded perfectly—they were in a sense the same thing. In draft notes written around this time on 'movement in animals', Harvey again described the heart as the 'general and ruler', which 'governs the whole body' like a 'King, the first and highest authority in the state'.

Charles shared his physician's vision of the consanguinity of physiology and politics. When Harvey brought before him the young nobleman with the exposed heart, the monarch considered the beating organ from a physiological point of view; but then he immediately, and effortlessly, segued to politics, the microcosm offering an obvious moral for the body politic. 'I wish', he told the unfortunate young man, 'I could perceive the thoughts of some of my nobilities' hearts as I have seen your heart.'

Harvey's comparison of the King and the heart to 'the Sun' was equally conventional. He was one of many writers of the period who celebrated England's 'sun king', one poet hailing Charles as 'A little living Sunne, Sonne of the living Light'. Renaissance astronomers also saw the links between heart, sun and king. In the middle of the sixteenth century Nicolaus Copernicus described the sun as 'seated on his Royal throne, guiding his family of planets as they circle round him'; his intellectual heir, the German Johannes Kepler, evoked an omnipotent sun, 'king of the planets for his motion, heart of the world for his power'. When these stargazers looked up at the heavens, they saw what the metaphorical links of their language and thought processes prompted them to see: a sun-heart, the king of the cosmos, swam effortlessly into their ken.

The analogy between the heart and the sun was one of many comparisons current in the seventeenth century between the microcosm, or the little world of man's body, and the macrocosm that was the universe. In one of his poems John Donne described man's body as 'an epitome of God's great booke'—the world.

Within Harvey's and Donne's intellectual horizon, everything was intimately related to, and imitated, everything else. The body was attuned to the harmony of the heavens. Being born under a particular star sign heavily influenced a man's character; the celestial spheres governed his external anatomy, the planets acted on his body fluids and internal organs. Bloodletting anywhere near the heart would only be successful if performed under the sign of Leo, which exercised a powerful influence over that noblest, lion-like organ. Astrology also informed the diagnosis and prognosis of a disease.

The humours of the body were the equivalents of the four elements. Hot and moist blood was like the air and tended to be produced in spring and childhood; hot and dry choler, which corresponded with fire, was associated with summer and youth. Diseases caused by short-term imbalances in the humours were treated in the appropriate season, bloodletting being most effective in spring.

God had composed the cosmos into one great 'chain of being'. At its zenith the almighty architect sat enthroned above a host of angels and demons; the stars and planets, arranged below these spirits, revolved audibly, producing sweet melodies. These heavenly bodies provided man, who was next in the chain, with a 'majestical roof fretted with golden fire'. Man was followed by the animal, vegetable and mineral orders, who, like him, inhabited the earth.

Every link in the chain resembled its immediate neighbour. There were also a million 'correspondences' between entities separated by some distance within the hierarchy. Being the noblest examples of their kind, the sun, the heart, the king, the lion and gold were regarded as alike. Natural histories listed all the correspondences between a particular animal and various entities in the natural, celestial and artificial worlds. These correspondences formed an essential part of the animal's being; their identification was one of the ends of natural philosophy.

Looking at entities within the microcosm and macrocosm, Donne and Harvey saw correspondences, similarities and hidden sympathies everywhere. In his lectures Harvey remarked on the kinship between kidneys and beans, 'hence, *kidney beenes*'; he also told his audience that the human spleen resembled 'the tongue of an Ox' and 'the sole of the foot.'

Understanding and harnessing the power of correspondences was one of the aims of the physician; another was identifying what, in Donne's words:

> the influence of the stars may be
> Imprisoned in an Hearbe, or Charme, or Tree,
> And doe by touch, all which the stars could doe.

As certain herbs and plants corresponded with the organs of the body, it was believed they might help cure them. Borage resembled the eye so it was used to treat that organ, while walnuts were believed to heal a wounded or troubled brain. There were infinite invisible sympathies between objects too: the magnet attracted iron because it was akin to it; the moon controlled its sister the sea. These hidden powers could be exploited for medical ends. To heal a battle wound, ointment was sometimes applied to the weapon that caused it rather than to the wound itself.

The seventeenth-century mind was famously described as an ocean where each kind, or entity within the natural world, 'Does straight his own resemblance find' within the chain of being. Praised by some admirers for ingenuity in devising experiments, and for the clarity of his observations, Harvey was even more famous among his contemporaries as a man 'fertile in recognizing resemblances', and as a philosopher of extraordinary imagination whose 'fancy' often 'outran' his reason. His mind moved in bold metaphorical leaps, and to freewheeling associative rhythms, identifying correspondences as it went. He described muscles in the human body as variously round, square, triangular, flat, hollow, long, narrow, short or fat; as such, they could, he argued, be 'likened analogously to a lizard, a mouse, a pear [or] a scalene'. Working together, muscles became 'masons, bricklayers, carpenters' who 'build the house' of the body, or 'musicians, bass, treble' in a performance where 'some sing, some dance, some act'.

Modern eyes see singularity and difference between objects in the world, and within the human body, believing this to be the only way of establishing 'facts' concerning them. In contrast Harvey and his contemporaries saw similarities, analogies and sympathies. As we do not believe in a 'chain of being' today, the identification of correspondences within it is no longer regarded as a valid form of knowledge. Yet as that mental act was believed to bring power in Harvey's period—the possibility, say, of harnessing the hidden sympathy between entities for medical purposes—it was certainly as 'real' and 'true' a variety of knowledge for Harvey's age as the discerning of the 'facts of nature' is for our own.

As Harvey scribbled away at his treatise, references to the macrocosm–microcosm issued effortlessly from his quick-moving pen. The parallel between the blood vessels and rivers offered itself to his consciousness. From the left ventricle of the heart, Harvey wrote, blood is 'diffused through the arteries' just as 'our Thames falls into the sea'. Galen had likened the movement of blood in the vessels to the ebb and flow of the sea, following the pattern of the tide, but for Harvey the dark liquid moved sure and fast like the Thames that flowed in front of the Ludgate house in which he wrote.

Memories associated with gushing water flooded into Harvey's mind. He recalled Padua, the *città d'acque* (city of water), with its forty-two stone bridges, beneath which the water of the Bacchigliano river flowed free, dividing into two and carving up the city's beating heart before joining the River Brenta east of the city. As a student, Harvey had followed the river's eastward course on his tramps into the 'fertile and spacious plaine' of the Veneto. One day, his ramblings had taken him to 'the waters of Spa, or the so-called waters of "Our Lady" in the Paduan countryside'; he recalled the occasion now as he sat at his writing table. The mineral spring, fed by the accumulation of rain-water beneath the earth, welled up from its underground reservoir to the surface: the 'water, permeating through the earth's substance', giving rise to bubbling 'streams'. In exactly the same way, Harvey wrote in his treatise, 'the blood permeates from the right ventricle through the lungs into the [pulmonary vein] and the left ventricle'. Once again, Harvey was tapping into a reservoir of cultural commonplaces here. In a poem which refers to the heart, Donne evokes 'streames like veines', that 'run through earth's every part'. In a sermon he declared that: 'Man consists of more pieces, more parts, than the world', before going on to argue that 'if all the veines in our bodies were extended to Rivers' they would overwhelm the terrestrial sphere.

Harvey's analogy was not merely a quaint illustration used for illustrative purposes, but an authentic form of knowledge. Just as Harvey held that one could learn about the heart by observing the king's position and function within the commonwealth, he also believed that knowledge of the movement of river water might help him understand the flow of the blood within the body. Leonardo da Vinci actually devised river experiments in a bid to shed light on the motion of the blood. We do not know whether Harvey made similar investigations, but he certainly shared the vision of the intertwined microcosm and macrocosm that inspired them.

✄ Essay 6 ℞

The landscape of Harvey's imagination (II): Perfect circles

THROUGH HIS QUEST, Harvey's imagination had run in, and on, circles. At a certain point in his treatise he describes the moment when he had started to entertain the idea that blood might have a 'circular motion'. Some paragraphs later, he places the idea within the context of the macrocosm. 'Blood travels swiftly through the whole body and nourishes . . . all its parts, truly no otherwise than the superior luminaries, the Sun and the Moon, give life to this inferior world by their continuous circular motions.'

The raw 'data' perceived by Harvey's eyes was realigned by his mind into the shape of a circle. Observing the snakes and slugs that formed part of his private menagerie, Harvey saw how they progressed inside their glass jars by 'a circumvolutary movement, bending themselves into arcs of a circle', through sinuous motion or undulation. Dogs were associated in his mind with the figure too, their forms in movement making 'a picture of a circle'.

During his vivisections of animals Harvey noticed how their muscles often 'worked by turns' or 'together' to produce in the limbs of the body, 'a circular movement'. 'The muscles and the ligaments together', he mused, 'push and pull and so cause movement in a circle.' He also discerned 'the phenomenon of circular movement' in the almost 'imperceptible movements' of the muscles themselves, which 'are like the turning of a wheel', tracing a 'spiral or a circular line'.

In the seventeenth century the circle was the symbol of perfection. Man's death, declared Donne, may end 'one circle' of life, yet it also opens another: 'for immortality, and eternity is a circle too; not a circle where two points meet, but a Circle made at once; This life is a Circle, made with a Compasse, that passes from point to point; That life is a Circle stamped with a print, an endlesse, and perfect Circle . . . Of this Circle, the Mathematician is our great and good God.' The phrase 'perfect circle' reverberates through the poetry of the period; the author George Chapman uses the adjective 'circulare' as a synonym for 'perfect'.

Circular forms were considered perfect because, as George Puttenham wrote in *The Art of English Poesy* (1589), they have 'no speciall place of beginning nor end,' and so 'beareth a similitude with God and eternitie'. What better way for the natural philosopher to celebrate God's creation, and to bear witness that it was His handiwork, than by discovering within it endless circles and circular patterns?

Harvey was by no means the only intellectual to do so. Astronomers traced circular patterns in the skies. In 1543 Copernicus famously hypothesized that all the planets, including the earth, 'circled' around the sun. 'The idea seemed absurd', he admitted, both to common sense, and also in terms of the sensory evidence available to him; yet 'as others before me had been permitted to assume certain circles in order to explain the motions of the stars' he believed that he would be readily permitted to entertain his circular theory.

Kepler believed that the motion of planets *had* to be perfectly circular, the planets being visible symbols of God's perfection. Yet observation seemed to suggest that the path of the celestial bodies was actually elliptical, as Kepler was eventually (and reluctantly) forced to admit. Even then, however, the German astronomer felt compelled to invent an excuse to explain the discrepancy—the planets, he declared, must be partly composed of earth, and, being made of that impure material, they could not imitate exactly the 'beauty and nobleness of the circular form'.

William Gilbert (1544–1603) was the English pioneer of the study of magnetism. A graduate of Cambridge, president of the College of Physicians, and personal physician to Elizabeth I, Gilbert began his investigations by constructing a magnet in the shape of a globe. He chose the spherical form because it agreed 'best with the earth' and was 'the most perfect'. The fruit of Gilbert's researches was his 1600 magnum opus *De Magnete* (*On the Magnet*), in which he suggested that the lodestone was a microcosm of the earth, as it moved according to 'the earth's position, whereby it adjusts itself to the earth's law'—that is, in a 'circular motion'. Gilbert would conclude that the earth itself was a great spherical magnet with iron at its heart.

Robert Fludd (1574–1637) was a fellow of the College of Physicians and a keen anatomist, who attended the demonstrations Harvey gave in support of his circulation theory. The pair became 'special friends' and intellectual allies, with Harvey citing Fludd in his lectures and writings. A gentleman-born, and an influential member of the medical establishment, Fludd was socially reputable and intellectually respected, King James himself sometimes summoning Fludd to his presence to discuss natural and mystical philosophy.

For Fludd was also a hermetic philosopher, adept in astrology and alchemy—by no means uncommon intellectual pursuits in the period (Fludd's alchemical activities were in fact encouraged by the Privy Council which gave him a patent to produce steel in his alchemical laboratory). In the hermetic arts, which derived from the ancient occult tradition and which flourished throughout Europe in Harvey's period, God was represented as 'a circle whose circumference is everywhere and whose centre is nowhere'. In

Utriusque cosmi, the vast and labyrinthine history of the microcosm and the macrocosm Fludd wrote in the mid-1620s (while Harvey was researching his treatise), divine circles and circular processes abound. When God first breathed his divine spirit into the air to create the world, Fludd tells us that it formed a 'circular motion'. In imitation of that great creating 'circle of divine wind', the sun now moves, according to Fludd, in circular motion in the sky.

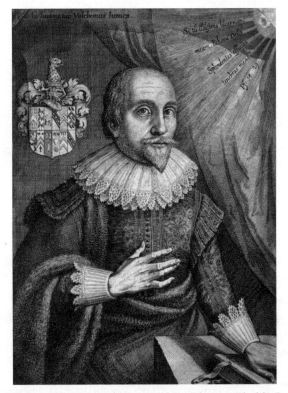

Portrait of Robert Fludd, the fifth son of Sir Thomas Fludd. On the right we see the circular sun, a symbol which features throughout his esoteric writings.

The motto of hermetic philosophers such as Fludd was 'as it is above, so it is below': what occurred in the heavens also happened on earth, and what was true for the macrocosm must hold for the microcosm also. In *Utriusque cosmi* Fludd applied these ideas to the specific question of the passage of the blood within the human body. According to him, God continually breathes spirit into the air where it forms a 'circle of divine wind'; this wind is distributed by the sun to the earth in 'circulatory air currents'. These currents are then taken into the microcosmic body via the lungs. From there they are drawn up into the heart, which sends them out as 'divine aerial spirit' within the arterial blood, to distribute invigorating spiritual life force throughout the body. The heart thus imitates the sun in its shape and workings, being 'the sun of the microcosm'. In pulsation, it acts like the distributing sun, sending spiritualized blood and vital heat around the body. The blood flows in a broadly 'circular' fashion, in imitation of the fiery sun in orbit and the winds that do its bidding. The blood's movement is also circular in the sense that its journey is endlessly repeated, just as the sun rises and sets daily.

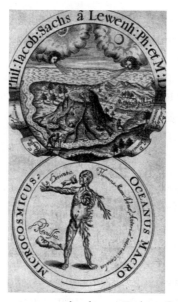

Fludd's ideas were common to the hermetical tradition. Here, in the frontispiece to an esoteric seventeenth-century text, we see an image of the correspondence between the cardiovascular system and the elements of the macrocosm.

Giordano Bruno, the occult philosopher burned at the stake for heresy in Rome in 1600, had argued along similar lines to Fludd. 'Spiritual life force is effused from the heart into the whole of the body', he declared, 'and flows back from the latter to the heart . . . following the pattern of a circle.' The Italian also speculated that 'the blood which in the animal body moves in a circle' does so 'continually and most rapidly'.

Bruno arrived at these conclusions from the first principle that the circle is the figure of divinity. As man partook of the divine, his blood must perforce move in the only shape that was continual, constant and perfect. According to Bruno, the human soul, endowed with divine intelligence, actively *chose* the ideal form of a circular pathway for the blood within the body, just as the heavens and the weather elected to trace that shape in the firmament through their movements. The body, like the universe, was intelligent and alive.

Ideas relating to the circular movement of the blood were also current in more conventional philosophical and medical traditions. When the ancients contemplated the microcosm of their anatomy and attempted to describe the movement of their blood, they often used analogies of the circle and circulation. Plato thought that the 'depletion and repair' of the body's organs by the blood was a cyclical process, its movement imitating the motion of the heavens—that is, it resembled a sort of 'circuit'.

Plato's student, Aristotle, was obsessed with circular patterns, perceiving the outline of that figure throughout the universe. 'When water is transformed into air', he wrote, outlining the meteorological 'cycle', 'air into fire, and fire back into water, we say that the "coming-to-be" has completed the circle, because it reverts again to the beginning.' This perpetual 'coming-to-be' was ubiquitous, for 'all things under the heavens', he declared, 'are moved in a circle'. Generation in nature, the process of seed-foetus-child-adult-seed, was thus an eternal 'cycle'—a 'kind of continuous regeneration' that perpetuated the species.

Given Harvey's propensity to see circles everywhere, and his conviction that 'the body imitates the harmony that reigns in the celestial heavens'; and bearing in mind the anatomical, philosophical and hermetic ideas in the intellectual air around him, it may have been with sense of familiarity and even inevitability that he suddenly saw, at a certain point in his researches, the movement of the blood within the body as perfectly, divinely, circular.

Aristotle's description of the meteorological cycle may have been especially important for Harvey, just as it had been crucial for William Gilbert's investigations into magnetism. Twenty years previously, Gilbert found an Aristotelian analogy for the globe's 'circular motion' in the perpetual movement of the 'humours of the earth, poured out through springs, and returned to its interior by gravitation'. The motion of the blood, Harvey now wrote in his treatise, 'we may call circular, after the same manner that *Aristotle* sayes that the rain and the air do imitate the motion of the superiour bodies. For the earth being wet, evaporates by the heat of the Sun, and the vapours being rais'd aloft are condens'd and descend in showers and wet the ground, and by this means here are generated, likewise, tempests, and the beginnings of meteors, from the circular motion of the Sun and his approach and removal. So in all likelihood, it comes to pass in the body, that all the parts are nourished, cherished, and quickned with blood, which is warm, perfect, vaporous, full of spirit, and, that I may so say, alimentative.' Harvey thus compares the perpetual cycle of evaporation and condensation in the macrocosm to the heart's recurrent revivification of the exhausted venous blood.

When Harvey meditated upon the heart's concoction of the blood, he found other analogies for it too. 'In the parts', he wrote, 'the blood is refrigerated, and made as it were barren, from thence it returns to the heart, to recover its perfection, and there again by naturall heat, powerfull and vehement, it is melted, and is dispens'd again through the body, being fraught with spirits.' In other words the liquid was 'circulated' in the heart, in the alchemical sense of being distilled.

The word 'circulation' was used by alchemists as a synonym for the distillation of a liquid for the purposes of refinement. George Ripley's long poem *Compound of Alchymy* taught its readers 'how to make / Of all thine Elements a perfect circulation'. The vessel in which alchemical distillation took place was commonly known as a 'circulatory', an English word coined in 1559. It is within a circulatory that Subtle, a character in Ben Jonson's popular satirical play *The Alchemist* (1610), sets 'the liquor Mars to circulation'.

In his Lumleian lectures, Harvey had explained how all the major organs 'circulated' liquids. 'Just as by chemistry', he had remarked, 'divers Heates, vessels, furnaces draw away the phlegme, fermentate and prepare, circulate and perfect; soe Nature has devised [the organs to] act as alchemists by means of different furnaces and heats'. In his treatise on the heart, he now presented the organ as an alchemical circulatory.

In making this comparison, Harvey may have been influenced by Fludd. Just as the alchemist aimed to perfect earth's substances, most famously endeavouring to transmute base metal into gold, so too, Fludd had claimed, did the heart perfect the impure blood by means of 'circulation'. Alternatively, Harvey may have derived the idea from the Italian anatomist Andreas Cesalpino, a student of Colombo, who had made the same parallel in his writings on the function of the heart, which were published between 1571 and 1602.*

---

* Alchemical circulatory movements continued to provide leitmotifs for the works of natural philosophers throughout the seventeenth century. At the end of the period the alchemist and astronomer Isaac Newton suggested that 'The whole frame of Nature may be nothing but various Contextures of some certain aethereall Spirits or vapours condens'd as it were by prae-cipitation . . . and after condensation wrought into various formes, at first by the immediate hand of the Creator, and ever since by the power of Nature . . . for nature is a perpetual circulatory worker, generating fluids out of solids, and solids out of fluids.'

Yet in truth Harvey could have taken the notion from anywhere, as it was embedded within the language in which he thought. It is surely significant that around this time, many words relating to circles, circular patterns and circulation entered everyday parlance, along with the alchemical terms such as 'circulation'. 'Circuit' ('to go or move in a circuit') was first used in 1611; the adjective 'circuitous' came into being in around 1620; 'circulator' (i.e. 'he who or that which circulates') entered the language in 1607, while 'circularity' had been employed since the 1580s. The currents of the English language undoubtedly carried Harvey towards his theory.

Whatever his influences—conscious, or absorbed by a sort of linguistic and cultural osmosis—one thing is clear from the account Harvey now committed to paper. He had first *imagined* that blood 'might' have a circular motion and then afterwards, during trials and further mental elaborations, 'found it true'—the idea, the inspiration, preceded the experiments. We are a long way here from the Baconian empiricist, patiently constructing a theory from a myriad of facts, beloved of most nineteenth-(and twentieth-)century Harvey biographers. We are in fact much closer to the nineteenth-century poet, William Blake, who wrote 'What is now proved was once only imagined.'

৺৪ Essay 7 ৶৵

Everyday influences on
Harvey's theory

As HARVEY TOILED away on his opus, images of the city around him crowded into his mind, just as the sounds of London must have filtered into the room in which he sat at his task. His writing was open to quotidian, as well as to intellectual and cultural, influences; the *genius loci* of seventeenth-century London presided over his treatise.

In one section of his work, he recalled having gazed on, fascinated, as the butchers in and around Smithfield went about their bloody business. 'In killing an oxe', he noticed, the butchers 'cut the jugular arteries', while the animal was still alive, in order to 'drain out the whole mass of blood in less than a quarter of an hour, emptying all the vessels'. This was evidence, Harvey claimed, that the heart muscle, in forceful contraction, evacuated blood from the body. If the butchers made the mistake of knocking the ox dead with a blow to the head, it was impossible, he noted, 'to draw from [the ox] above half the mass of blood'.

We may think of Harvey hurrying through London's maze-like streets during the period in which he penned his treatise, observing everything, allowing numberless details of city life to permeate his prose. In notes written around this time he described the child on Holborn Bridge who had a beard only 'on the one cheek'; a beggar behind Covent Garden with a hernia 'bigger than his belly'. He evoked the boys 'leaping' and 'hoping' as they played football in Smithfield, along with the passing gentry and tradesmen who gathered round to watch their boisterous delights.

Harvey plundered the city's streets of imaginative analogies for microcosmic features and processes. One day on his rambles he came across a horse drinking water at one of the city's pools, and noticed how its neck muscles made a curious sound as they drew up the liquid. 'The water is sup'd down into the belly,' he wrote afterwards, the process 'yielding a certain noise and pulse. In the same way,' he reflected, 'whilst some portion of the blood is drawn out of the veins into the arteries, there is a beating which is heard within the breast.'

In Harvey's writings, the city itself is transformed into a vast body. On one occasion his professional duties took him from St Paul's Cathedral to Leadenhall Market. As he made the short journey he noticed that though he was walking down a single long thoroughfare ('from Powles to leden hale one way'), the roads were called 'buy many names [such] as cheape powtry [Cheapside and Poultry]'. This reminded him of the way the intestine formed a single channel within the body, but was comprised of sections differing in 'substance, shape and name', such as the duodenum, colon and rectum.

The city-body metaphor, which is at least as old as Plato, was popular in Harvey's period. London was often compared to a gluttonous body 'grown great' with overpopulation and overindulgence. Thomas Dekker, an extravagant and popular prose stylist of the period, 'anatomized' London's sick and 'bloated body' in his writings; John Stow, the great Elizabethan London topographer, divides the city into separate parts in *The Survey of London* (1598), as though conducting a detailed dissection.

If London became a body in Harvey's mind, it was also transformed into a heart. Here too, he drew on a commonplace of the time. The 'lion-hearted' Henry VIII had called London the 'heart of the

Kingdom'. The Jacobean dramatist Thomas Middleton noted that it stood 'in the middle of the land', thereby occupying 'as in the body, the heart's place'. London was, it was said, the first organ in the commonwealth to receive life, from the presence of the king and his government there; by the same logic it would also be the last organ to die. Dekker feared that the city's death was imminent, Westminster, the city's administrative 'heart', having become attenuated by greed. That organ was now so enfeebled, he complained, that it was unable to carry out its function of governing—it could no longer 'stirr uppe' the city's 'bloud' and so maintain its health.

Harvey's theory was unusual within the anatomical and physio- ogical tradition, as it emphasized the rapidity of the flow of the blood around the body. The etymology of *cor*, the Latin word for heart, was, Harvey believed, *currere*—something which 'perpetually runs' or is in 'constant motion'. In evoking the quickness of the blood's flow, and the rapid throbbing of the heart, Harvey's prose resembles that of social commentators who described the traffic coursing through the veins of England's capital city. The flow of people and four-wheeled traffic within late Elizabethan London was unremitting, as Stow pointed out. There were now numberless 'cars, drays, carts, and coaches—more than hath been accustomed . . . the world runs on wheels with many whose parents were glad to go on foot.'

Yet any obstruction to the frenetic flow of people and traffic was regarded by the city authorities as unwelcome and unhealthy. London's governors compelled citizens to keep the streets unblocked; they were obliged to clean the roads in front of their houses, and were forbidden to deposit dung there. Large-scale traffic projects were also undertaken. Newgate had, according to Stow, been built with the express purpose of facilitating the flow of traffic within the city, allowing 'men and cattle, with all manner of carriages, to pass more directly from Aldegate, through West Cheape by Pauls on the north side; and from thence to any part westward over Oldbourne bridge, or turning into Smithfielde, to any part North'.

Harvey saw the traffic flowing freely beneath Newgate as he passed it on his weekly journey to and from St Bartholomew's Hospital in Smithfield.

London was the beating heart of England so far as trade was concerned. The city, as one seventeenth-century economic commentator put it, 'gathered commodities' from the provinces and from foreign lands, then 'dispersed them from thence into the country'. As such, London was 'the source' and 'spring' of all 'rivers of trade' in England: 'all the weight of [English] trade falles to this centre, & comes within the circuit of this circle'.

Harvey knew all about the rapid and constant flow of trade within the kingdom (from circumference to centre, and then back to circumference again). Five of his six brothers were well established in business. Daniel Harvey, the fourth of Thomas Harvey's sons, purchased and then transported all the tin mined in Devon and Cornwall to the London market. He also imported cloth, silk and 'black velvett' from Aleppo, Constantinople, Genoa and Hamburg. In the English capital he sold these goods for a tidy profit to men who in turn distributed them throughout the country. Daniel became wealthy, and with money came renown: he was one of the dedicatees of Lewis Roberts' popular manual of trade *The Merchants Mappe of Commerce* (1638). Interestingly, William Harvey was another dedicatee, which suggests that he too was interested in trade, at least from a theoretical point of view; perhaps he dabbled in it also, speculating in commodities and on the money markets.

In Harvey's treatise, the heart is described as gathering and dispensing blood within the body, via and the veins and the arteries, in the same way that London collected goods and money from the country, only to return them there. Harvey argued that for health to be preserved, there had to be a constant 'activity' of the heart, as well as a 'vigorous circulation of the blood'. On no account should either the organ or the liquid become 'sluggish', 'congested', 'slowed' or 'constricted'. This is strongly reminiscent of the recommendations made by contemporary economists concerning trade within the kingdom.

Medieval London had been serviced by a series of rivers and brooks. According to Stow, Walbrooke ran 'through the midst of the city, serving the heart thereof'. There was also a 'bourn, watering the part in the east', as well as a network of fountains, wells and pools. 'Besides all which, they had in every street and lane of the city divers fresh springs; and after this manner was the city served with sweet and fresh waters.'

These wells and waters had diminished by Stow's and Harvey's time, and had also become clogged up with refuse which typically included 'dead Hogges, Dogges, Cats, Beasts' guts'. Recognizing that a free circulation of fresh water was essential to the city's health, the authorities sought 'other means to supply the want.' These included an intricate network of cisterns, fountains and conduits—a word generally used to denote the lead pipes that carried water to the fountains, but which was sometimes used as a synonym for the fountain itself.

As clean water was precious, illegal attempts were often made to divert it from the main pipes. The College of Physicians may have been among the offenders. The city authorities complained about a 'quill [a pipe the width of a swan's neck] of water taken by the College, which had been fraudulently cutt by [its] plummer'. They declared that the fellows either had to prove their right to the quill, or would have to construct at their own cost a pipe that would provide twenty-four gallons of water per day along with a cistern large enough to receive it. The college reacted angrily to the accusations, and its trusty delegate William Harvey was dispatched to the Star Chamber to settle the dispute. In investigating the affair, Harvey must have learned a fair deal about the city's waterworks.

There was a cistern close to Harvey's home in Ludgate, the water being carried there by lead pipes from Paddington. It was, according to Stow, 'garnished with images of St Christopher on the top, and angels lower down, with sweet sounding bells before them, where-upon, by an engine placed, the divers hours of the day and night chimed such an hymn as was appointed'. 'The poor' of the area drank from it while rich families, such as the Harveys, used the water to 'dress their meats'—indicating its indifferent quality.

'London', an observer wrote, has 'good veins in her body . . .[and] good blood in her Veins, by those many Aqueducts, Conduits, and conveyances of fresh waters, to serve for all uses.' This common comparison transplanted the ancient parallel between rivers and the blood vessels to a new artificial context. John Donne, ever a conduit for the spirit of his age, had spoken in a sermon of the 'conduits and cisterns of the body' which house its blood.

Harvey used the metaphor to great effect in his writing, comparing the heart and its vessels to the man-made waterways within the city. The vena cava, he remarked, opened 'into the heart just as into a cistern'—suggesting that the blood poured into it, like water from lead pipes. The organ indeed functioned, according to Harvey, exactly like one of the 'fowntayns [and] conduits', which he saw all around him.

Diverting the course of a river, or conveying water via lead pipes to cisterns, was often compared to a natural process, one commentator likening the pipes and conduits of the city to 'rivulets' and 'springs'. Yet the capital's water system was of course an 'ingenious fabrick', as Stow called it, a 'Herculean work' of artifice, heavily reliant on mechanical devices.

In 1582 the Dutch hydraulic engineer Peter Morice had built a huge waterwheel on the north arch of London Bridge. A series of water pumps attached to it squirted a jet of water as high as the steeple of the nearby Church of St Magnus Martyr. These pumps propelled the water from the wheel towards Laurence Poultney, where a fountain was constructed. A similar device was built in the sixteenth century at Bygot House, just to the west in Queen Hithe, a stone's throw from Harvey's home. Bevis Bulmar had, Stow recorded, constructed an engine in that building 'for the conveying and forcing [i.e. pumping] of Thames water to . . . the middle and west parts of the city'.

Pumps had been used in Europe for centuries to drain and irrigate arable land, as well as to raise water out of mines. During Harvey's lifetime, they started to be built in the 'engins' used by firefighters. In the early seventeenth century John Bates described, in his *Mysteries of Nature and Art*, one such device 'which being placed in water will cast the same with violence on high'. In Bates' homely English, the valves inside this pump are referred to as 'clacks'—pieces of 'Leather nailed over any hole having a peece of Lead to make it lie close, so that ayre or water in any vessel may thereby bee kept from going out'. Clacks were built into wind and water bellows as well as water pumps; opened by the upward or downward movement of wind or water, the purpose of the clack was to regulate its flow.

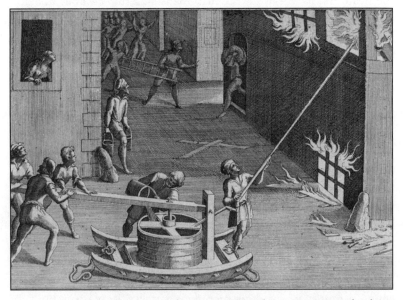

Fire pumps shown in Salomon de Caus' 1615 volume *Les raisons des forces mouvantes*. 'There are two valves in the pump,' de Caus wrote, 'one below to open when the handle is lifted up and shut when it is down, another to open to let out the water.'

As Harvey penned his treatise, his mind moved in a perpetual process of analogy, seeking out similarities, sympathies and corre-spondences between the microcosm and the macrocosm. Sometimes, and probably without any particular intention or philosophical consideration in mind, Harvey likened the insides of the body to artificial devices. Thus, discussing the movement of the heart, Harvey first compared it to the action of the neck muscles of a horse as it swallowed water. To elucidate the idea further he then used the parallel of 'that mechanical device fitted to firearms in which, on pressure of a trigger, a flint falls and strikes and advances the steel, a spark is evoked and falls upon the powder, the powder is fired and the flame leaps inside and spreads, and the ball flies out'.

While scribbling away, Harvey's rapid train of thought, and the links of his language, carried him irresistibly to idea that the heart worked like a set of water bellows. 'From the structure of the heart', he wrote, 'it is clear that the blood is constantly carried to the lungs and into the aorta as by two clacks of a water bellows to rayse water.' Harvey was suggesting that the heart's valves (the 'little doors' located at the base of the pulmonary artery and aorta) act like clacks, preventing the flow of blood back into the heart and facilitating its journey out of the organ.

Harvey must have seen these 'clacks' in action in water or wind bellows. In the description of the lungs he made during his Lumleian lectures, he had remarked that 'respiration occurs in two ways' as 'in two sides of bellows; the upper part in the bellows is where *ye clack*'. This parallel between the valve and the clack in a set of bellows was novel; so too was the implication that the heart was a sort of machine that maintained pressure within the blood vessels. Tradition taught that the arteries had an active 'pulsative force', but to Harvey the blood vessels were passive, like the lead pipes that conveyed pumped water into London's cisterns. The heart was the machine that carried out all the work.

And indeed, perhaps Harvey was already thinking of the heart as a kind of pump. 'When you cut off an arterie', he would write some years later, clarifying the ideas of his treatise, 'you observe that the flux' of the blood is 'continuall; though it be sometimes nigher, sometimes further.' He compared this to 'water' that 'by the force and impulsion of a spout, is driven aloft through pipes of lead . . . [with] all the forcings of the Engine', which was continual though of increasing and decreasing 'vehemency'. Harvey probably had in mind here a water pump such as that designed by Bevis Bulmar. On another occasion, when he described the same phenomenon, he seems to have been thinking of a fire engine. The 'blood spurts out' of the artery, he wrote, 'as if spurted out from a syringe or piston pump'.

Following the Greek philosopher Heraclitus, William Harvey believed that the immortal gods were present everywhere, which was to say that 'nature is nowhere wont to reveal her secrets more openly than where she shows faint traces of herself away from the beaten track'. Important lessons could be learned from apparently inconsequential objects and events; inspiration could be found in everything, including the latest developments in trade and technology.

The city around Harvey fed and fired his imagination as he wrote; London got under his skin, and permeated his blood vessels. Its rush and push entered his head and the relentless and repetitive rhythms of his prose. Always 'hott-headed', according to a friend, Harvey's 'thoughts working would many times keep him from sleeping'. When his rapid reflections tortured him with insomnia, Harvey would 'rise out of Bed and walk about his Chamber in his Shirt'. At other times he paced round and round, tracing circles on the roof of his London house. Harvey's mind was synchronized with London time; if his thoughts never slept, neither did the city ever find complete rest. Even in the quietest hours, Harvey saw activity in the street as he gazed down from the rooftops—drunken revellers wandering home, shouting 'knave, rogue, coxcomb' at each other; horses and carts bringing produce up from the country to London's markets; servants rising before the sun.

And if Harvey was a man who discovered inspiration in everything, then who is to say that he did not tap into that reservoir of personal memories, which no doubt filled his mind on sleepless nights, when he sat down to work on his treatise? At many earlier stages of his life, he had encountered a host of suggestive circular symbols and processes. There was the circulatory system of goods and letters that formed the basis of his father's business; Cambridge's circulatory river system (in the south, the Cam resembles the city's vena cava, bringing water, people and goods, to its beating heart; in the north the river turns into an aorta, carrying liquid away from the city); the circular botanical gardens and anatomical theatre at Padua; the images of religious hearts Harvey may have seen in the city's cathedral; and the circular disputations he had participated in there. There is also a suggestive symmetry between Harvey's idea of the blood's fast, continuous motion, and the perpetual movement of Harvey's body and mind, often remarked on by his friends.

Caius Court at Cambridge offered possible inspiration too, not only through its circulating air. In the court there was a pump which servants used for washing and from which the students drank. Pushing down hard on its metal handle generated enough pressure to draw water up through the valve or 'clack'. Even this simple device may have offered the shadow of a crucial suggestion to a mind so fertile in recognizing resemblances.

12. Publication and reception (1628–1650s): "'Twas beleeved . . . he was crack-brained'

THROUGHOUT 1627, HARVEY worked on his treatise, which he entitled *De motu cordis*. Opening with his discovery of the forceful systole and the cause of the arterial pulse, Harvey then evoked the surprise he felt when he realized that a vast amount of blood was ejected by the contracting heart into the aorta. This served as a prelude to the discussion of the pulmonary transit and to the announcement of the circulation theory. Harvey shaped his book into the form of an extended academic disputation: dedicating a chapter to a particular argument, he presented objections to it, before addressing each of them in turn. Having settled one issue to his satisfaction he then moved on to the next.*

---

* It seems likely that the architecture of the treatise is based on Harvey's private demonstrations to his colleagues. If that is the case, then it is difficult to separate the stage of 'showing' the theory from that of 'discoursing' on it in writing. Similarly, the earlier division between the solitary 'trying' of the theory, and the public 'showing' of it, is hazy. It is unlikely that Harvey completed, and fully 'tried', his theory in solitude before he began demonstrating it—although that is the way that I have presented it here, for the sake of narrative clarity. The completed theory was probably conceived and born in public, Harvey's fellow physicians playing the part of midwives as it emerged gradually, during disputations which spanned almost a decade.

Fashioning his impressive scholarly structure would have taken Harvey a great deal of time. It is likely that he went through several drafts before writing '*finis*' on the last notebook page. He then presumably made a fair copy from his 'foul papers' (as early drafts were called) which he sent off to his Frankfurt publisher, the Englishman William Fitzer. Harvey may have chosen Fitzer on the recommendation of Robert Fludd, one of the publisher's authors, who would advise his friends to publish 'beyond the seas' because authors did not have to pick up the reckoning for the publication costs there, as they often did in England. On the other hand, Harvey may have been prevailed upon by the College of Physicians to publish on the Continent, the fellows desiring not to draw too much attention, in England, to their implied endorsement of a book so thoroughly anti-Galenic.

The final manuscript draft Harvey dispatched to Fitzer seems to have been more foul than fair, however. When *De motu cordis* was eventually published in the autumn of 1628 at the price of six schillings two pfennigs, it included a loose leaf with 126 errata, which covered only half of the typographical errors contained in the sixty-eight-page book. Harvey's notoriously obscure hand was probably to blame, though Fitzer may have also been guilty of negligence. Other aspects of the book's production were shoddy: in a bid to keep costs down Fitzer printed it in tiny blunt type on low-quality paper, and dressed it in an economical binding. For the illustrations of Harvey's ligature experiments, the publisher (or the artist he employed) lifted without acknowledgement an image from Fabricius' book on the 'little doors' of the veins. Fitzer did, however, take the trouble to adorn the volume with a striking title page, dominated by his own insignia.

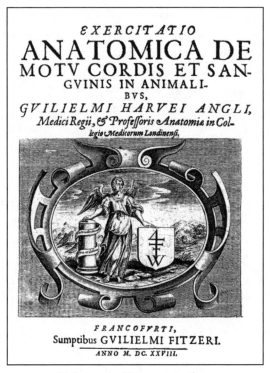

EXERCITATIO
ANATOMICA DE
MOTV CORDIS ET SAN-
GVINIS IN ANIMALI-
BVS,
GVILIELMI HARVEI ANGLI,
Medici Regii, & Professoris Anatomiæ in Col-
legio Medicorum Londinensi.

FRANCOFVRTI,
Sumptibus GVILIELMI FITZERI.
ANNO M. DC. XXVIII.

Title page of *De motu cordis*.

Harvey doubtless presented copies to its chief dedicatee
Charles I, as well as 'To the most Excellent and Ornate man D.
Argent, President of the College of Physicians in London', to
whom he had offered the book's secondary dedication. Harvey
distributed further copies among the fellows of the College of
Physicians.

On reading the book 'the grandees' of the college declared
themselves 'of the opposite judgment', their opposition being
widely considered as 'heavy enough', as one commentator put
it, 'to overlay (and so to stifle) the infant opinion by its authority'.
Most of the lesser fellows followed suit, expressing themselves
'against [Harvey's] Opinion'. Many 'wrote against him' too, using
the Galenic objections they had doubtless voiced during Harvey's

private demonstrations. They portrayed Harvey in print as the man who 'affected a vain commendation in dissection', 'dispraising and deriding' the 'Frogs and Serpents, Gnats, and other more inconsiderable creatures brought upon the stage' of the anatomist's prose.

They even went so far as to insinuate that Harvey had spent far too long among the dismembered corpses of animals, and meditating in the dark on abstruse theories, to be any longer fit to practise medicine. Even if his idea were cogent as an abstract philosophical theory (and they were reluctant to concede even this) it had, in their view, absolutely no relevance to medical treatment, which was, and always would be, Galenic in inspiration. 'In anatomy,' a fellow doctor wrote, 'and theoretic discoveries,' Harvey might 'pretend the precedency of all his Contemporaries.' Yet like 'others before or since who had arrived at great proficiency in dissecting; when concerned in [medical] Practice', Harvey was by no means 'gifted with the sagacity to know diseases . . . much less of curing them'.

This prejudice percolated down to Harvey's patients, one of whom became convinced that the doctor was 'too mutch governed by his Phantasy'. To have a physician abound in fantasy was, he thought, 'a very perilous thing . . . he should be governed only by his judgement'. As a result of this disposition to daydream, Harvey had, the patient complained, committed the folly of leaving behind 'the ancient rules, and set up new opinions for the maintenance of which' he was 'forced to great inconveniences . . . when brought into Practice'. Rumours of Harvey's eccentricity spread so widely that, as one friend wrote, it ''twas beleeved by the vulgar that he was crack-brained' and he 'mightily fell in his practice'.

While many physicians ridiculed Harvey, there were some who understood and praised his achievement. Soon after receiving a copy of the book, no doubt directly from Harvey himself, Robert Fludd penned a spirited defence of its central argument:

as we see that a single chord with its weight by a whole action
makes the minutes of the hour on the clock in the motion of one
circle or wheel . . . just so the vital spirit in the function of life
is moved in its vessels by the whole action of one spirit and in a
circle of wind. This seems to confirm exactly that notion and
opinion of the most grave William Harvey, skilful physician,
distinguished anatomist, and most experienced in the deepest
mysteries of philosophy, my dear compatriot and faithful colleague
. . . he clearly teaches the world in a certain little book of
his . . . both with argument drawn from philosophy's store and
with manifold ocular demonstration, that the movement of the
blood itself is circular. And why not, you cynics, when it is certain
that the spirit of life retains the impress both of the planetary
system and the zodiac? Thus, as the moon follows her unchanging
path, completing her journey in a month, she incites the spirit
of the blood to follow in a cyclical movement. Every seaman is
acquainted with the influence of the moon on wind and tide.
Why should she not exercise a similar influence in the 'microcosm'
of man?

This eulogy, translated from Fludd's baroque Latin, was published
in the fifth volume of his mystical work *Medicina Catholica* in 1629,
making it the very first defence of Harvey's theory to appear in
print.

Fludd's emphasis on the philosophical appeal of the circulation theory was typical. Many early readers of *De motu cordis*
were equally impressed by its broad arguments, and by its
dexterous application of pervasive and commonplace ideas and
metaphors to a specific physiological problem. The English
student of anatomy Roger Drake was excited by Harvey's 'ocular
demonstrations', yet what persuaded him of the power of the
theory was its philosophical and poetic coherence and sugges-
tiveness. He immediately grasped Harvey's parallel between

the blood flow and the meteorological cycle, and was equally taken by the comparison of the heart to an alchemical circulatory.

Anatomists enthusiastic about Harvey's theory described it as 'elegant' and 'neat'. It appeared to them to be 'simple, uniform, constant, harmonious', and, as it were, to rejoice in 'the simplicity and the order of nature'. It was iridescent with aesthetic appeal too, with one natural philosopher pronouncing it 'beautiful'. The theory also appeared to be eminently appropriate for the culture in which it was conceived. Supporters sensed that Harvey had become a lightning rod for the intellectual forces and language of his time, and had harnessed those powers brilliantly to animate anatomical ideas. His theory seemed orderly, graceful and comprehensible to them, precisely because it relied so heavily on common cultural ideas and metaphors. Emerging from the language and thought of its time, it appeared to 'make sense'.

The attractiveness was further enhanced by the fact that, deriving from the various languages of its culture (those of poetry, economics, politics, astronomy), it could be effortlessly translated back into those languages. This ensured its wider public dissemination. Astrologers such as the Italian Andrea Argoli championed the theory as a confirmation of the microcosm-macrocosm concept. Harvey, he declared, had discovered that blood imitates the perfect motion of the stars by travelling in circular fashion around man's body, that 'little version of the heavens'. Economists also enthusiastically adopted and adapted the theory. After Harvey, trade within England was often compared to blood 'which should flow circularly and freely' around the country. The great prose stylist Daniel Defoe marvelled at 'the circulation of trade within ourselves, where all the several manufactures move in a just rotation from several counties where they are made, to the city of London, as the blood in the body to the Heart; and from thence are dispers'd again'. Just as the economic analogy may have helped inspire

Harvey's theory, so in turn did the theory reinforce the parallel for economists.

Money would thenceforth be frequently likened to 'the blood' of the commonwealth, whose unimpeded circulation was necessary for 'the maintenance of life within the whole economy'. Engineers latched on to the idea too, creating machines driven by a 'perpetual circulatory pneumato-hydraulic motion'. Inspired by Harvey, Robert Fludd attempted to construct a 'perpetual motion machine' that powered itself by recycling water from a tank.

Poets made full and extravagant use of Harvey's inherently poetical idea, turning the circulation into a marvellous conceit. John Birkenhead wrote that just as:

> immortall Harvey's searching Brain
> Found the Red Spirit's Circle in each veyn . . .
> . . . So wit, the blood of Verse, in every line
> . . . proves its Circulation through all Arts.

Others discovered in the circulation of the blood an image of the entire universe: 'Thus we see almost everything', as one put it, 'Circling about as in a ring'; 'All things to Circulations owe / Themselves', wrote another, 'by which alone / They do exist.' Harvey's elaborate heart-sun-king metaphors were not lost on the poets either, one of them praising him as the anatomist who, after 'plunging steel into beasts', saw the heart as 'a sun breaking through the murky darkness' of their entrails.

After the publication of Harvey's theory, the word 'circulation' became ever more widely used. By the time of his death it was employed in countless new contexts, describing 'the passage of sap through the vessels of plants'; the 'transmission, or passage of goods from hand to hand'; the movement of anything that revolved or took a 'a circuitous course'; and the 'dissemination and publication' of literature or news. Having been prompted in part by the English language, the circulation theory in turn altered it forever.

The process by which ideas flowed between Harvey and the broader culture of his period can be compared to the functioning of the Harveian heart. The veins of culture and language conveyed blood-like ideas and words to his heart, which concocted them into a theory. The theory was then sent back out into the culture, through various languages, just as the arteries distributed blood throughout the body. There was a constant interchange and circulation of ideas and words between culture and theorist.

Despite the hostility of the medical world, the broad intellectual culture of the seventeenth century received Harvey's theory favourably because it was ripe for it—and, often, ripeness is all. It is surely no coincidence that numerous people 'happened' upon the idea of circulation at roughly this time. The anatomist Andreas Cesalpino anticipated virtually every element of Harvey's theory, even using the word 'circulation', albeit in exclusive reference to the chemical distillation of the blood. What the Italian lacked was the vision of the blood's rapid circular path which informed Harvey's work; had he discussed the matter with his fellow countryman Giordano Bruno, Cesalpino may very well have hit upon Harvey's idea. Bruno was convinced that blood moved continually and quickly in a circle within the body.

The English mathematician Walter Warner claimed, to his dying day, to have been the 'only begetter' of the circulation theory. Warner developed a theory of the alchemical 'circulation' of the blood independently of Harvey. The heart's function was broadly associated in his mind with contemporary hydraulic engineering, just as Harvey intuited that the heart worked like a kind of pump. Warner always maintained that he had communicated his thoughts on the subject to Harvey prior to the publication of *De motu cordis*, but there is no corroborating evidence for this. What is certain is that he was one of many thinkers who had an 'inkling' of the circulation before they had ever heard of William Harvey or his book.*

---

* Similar ideas often develop within a culture around the same time, perhaps chiefly because ideas are formulated in, and so shaped by, language. If we look back at the emergence of Charles Darwin's theory of the 'struggle for existence' we can see that it bears striking similarities to many other early and mid-nineteenth-century ideas such as Karl Marx's notion of the proletariat's triumphant progress through history, after periods of 'struggle' with the other classes, or Thomas Malthus' theory of exponential population creating intense competition and 'struggle' for human resources. It is also interesting to compare the *Origin of Species* with Samuel Smiles' famous *Self-Help* manual, a book which was published on the same day as Darwin's. Smiles celebrates the evolutionary benefits that 'struggle' (one of his favourite words) brings to 'nations as well as individuals'. 'It is hard to say', Smiles remarks, what evolutionary benefit 'northern nations owe to their . . . perennial struggle with [climatic and geological] difficulties the natives of sunnier climes know nothing of.' Growing out of its intellectual culture and language, Darwin's theory (like Harvey's) would, in turn, profoundly influence that culture and language, helping to shape the politics, philosophy, economics, literature and art of the coming age.

13. Dissemination and defence (1628–1636): 'He is a circulator!'

WHILE HIS CIRCULATION theory was bewildering physicians, and slowly capturing the imagination of poets and economists, Harvey had to fight against anatomical critics, on various intellectual fronts. The most hostile among them were Galenic anatomists such as James Primrose, who attacked Harvey's theory in his 1630 volume *Exercitationes, et animadversiones*. A young licentiate of the College of Physicians, Primrose aped Harvey by dedicating his book to both Dr Argent and Charles I, perhaps wishing to alert both Crown and college to the dangerous and radical implications of *De motu cordis*.

Primrose pandered to popular prejudice by scoffing at the menagerie of motley creatures Harvey experimented on; he also ridiculed Harvey's wild guesses concerning the quantity of blood leaving the contracting heart. Yet while Harvey's methods were laughable (according to Primrose) his theory was a deadly serious business: if his vicious attack on Galen proved successful, the whole temple of conventional anatomy and medical practice would topple to the ground. As Harvey offered nothing in place of this vast and venerable intellectual edifice, his aim was, Primrose suggested, to set anarchy loose on the intellectual world.

Harvey complained of the 'ill language' and 'incivility' of his critics. 'It cannot be eschewed', he retorted in *De Circulatione Sanguinis* (*Anatomical Exercitations concerning the Circulation of the Blood*), 'but dogs will bark and belch up their surfeits . . . but we must take a speciall care that they do not bite, nor infect us with their cruel madnesse, lest they should with their dogs teeth gnaw the very bones and principles of truth.' *Anatomical Exercitations* was an eloquent defence of the circulation theory addressed to Jean Riolan, professor of anatomy at the University of Paris and Galen's self-appointed representative on earth. Its publication in 1649, over twenty years after *De motu cordis*, indicates the extent and arduousness of Harvey's campaign to promote his theory. As part of that long crusade the Englishman penned and published various letters to other continental anatomists, and he occasionally gave public demonstrations.

As we have seen, one such demonstration took place in 1636 at Altdorf University, which Harvey visited during his travels on the Continent as a member of the diplomatic party Charles I sent to the Holy Roman Emperor Ferdinand II. After Harvey had concluded his lecture in the University's anatomy theatre, some students and members of the public pressed forward to get a better look at the dog he had vivisected. Others talked excitedly to their neighbours, exclamations of wonder filling the auditorium. Harvey was far more interested, however, in the reaction of his learned peers in the front row. In particular, he was curious to learn the opinion of a round-shouldered man with a thin white beard, dressed in the long black velvet robe of a professor. The professor was not much taller than Harvey, and roughly the same age. His name, as Harvey knew very well, was Caspar Hofmann, professor of medicine at the University of Altdorf, and doyen of the Nuremberg medical establishment.

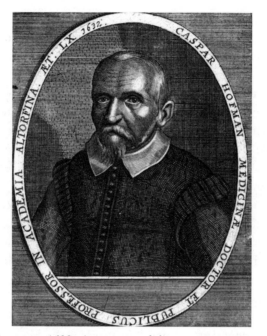

Caspar Hofmann in 1632. As mentor of the rising generation of German anatomists, Hofmann's favourable opinion was crucial to Harvey; the Altdorf demonstration may have been organized in a bid to win him over as an ally.

Harvey had reasons to be sanguine about his chances of securing Hofmann's assent and perhaps even his support for the circulation theory. The pair had been friends at the University of Padua, where they had studied under Fabricius, imbibing his Aristotelian vision of anatomy. After graduation Harvey and Hofmann had inhabited different worlds—the academy and the court—yet their intellectual development had followed broadly parallel lines with both maturing into brilliant and independent-minded anatomists. 'It is easy', Hofmann would remark to his students, apropos of traditional Galenic theory, 'to say that *these* [beliefs] *are ancient*, but it is not easy to know whether *they are true*.' Indeed Hofmann, like Harvey, publicly challenged a number of Galen's tenets; he also supported Colombo's theory of the transit of the blood across the lungs.

A number of Hofmann's pupils had already embraced Harvey's circulation theory, claiming that their professor's teaching had, as it were, cleared the way for, and prepared them to accept it. Several English critics had even accused Harvey of plagiarising Hofmann's ideas in *De motu cordis*. Harvey strenuously—and with much justice—denied the charge, although he was certainly familiar with Hofmann's writings. For his part, Hofmann knew *De motu cordis* inside out. And so the pair had remained in contact, through print and via third parties if not through personal letters, since their student days.

It was doubtless with a smile that Harvey now approached the front row of the Altdorf theatre and the friend he had last seen thirty-five years previously. 'I rejoice', he exclaimed, 'to see you, my dear old Hofmann, having looked forward to this meeting for so long. I could not in any way miss the chance of seeing, during this my European expedition, such a knowledgeable and upright man as yourself, a man whose friendly discourse used so to delight me in our student days in Italy.' 'My dear Harvey,' Hofmann replied, 'your kindness makes me not only your friend once again, but also your debtor.'

Pleasantries exchanged, Harvey turned the conversation to his theory, in the hope of a public endorsement. 'And, now that you have witnessed my demonstration, dear Hofmann,' he asked, 'pray give me your opinion of my theory of the circulation of the blood.' 'As I am your debtor', Hofmann responded, 'I will readily give you my opinion in payment of my debt. My hope is that you will receive it in the spirit in which it is offered—without a trace of ill will, but rather simply and sincerely.' The German's words may have unsettled Harvey; without doubt, they prepared him for criticism.

Hofmann offered his 'first objection' to the theory, in accordance with the format of an academic disputation. 'I must confess that I found it difficult to distinguish between the systole and diastole of the dog's heart—the heart beats too quickly for these movements to be identified by sight, and nothing incontrovertible can be established on the matter through observation. Anyone can argue that it is so, but it is another thing to demonstrate it.'

'I confess, my fair-minded Hofmann,' Harvey responded, 'how perplexing a matter this is, but I know what I have just seen with my eyes, and I believe you saw it too.' Although he was evidently unsatisfied by this, Hofmann turned to another objection: 'I would also like to learn from you Harvey, by what paths the blood goes out of the arteries and back into the veins? The vessels do not meet, nay, they end in flesh.'

'Learned Hofmann,' the Englishman answered, 'it must be that they pass indirectly through porosities in the flesh, or directly through anastomosis.' 'I must confess my bewilderment,' Hofmann countered, 'for I understand neither means.' 'I do not understand the matter yet clearly myself, my dear Hofmann,' Harvey replied, 'but the man who demonstrates the circulation is not to be dismissed simply because he does not know the routes and facilities in detail, for such enquiry comes later. Contradiction from such things is, if I may say so, for the sake of argument only.'*

Hofmann had grown imperious with age and with the eminence of his position; his importance, and the presence of a large and familiar audience, made him arrogant towards his old companion. 'Well, then,' he scoffed, 'let it be granted that these passages exist, unknown to so many preceding centuries, but now discovered by an Englishman, who admits that he cannot actually see them and does as yet not fully understand their workings.' The acerbic aside probably provoked laughter in an audience which enjoyed a piquant scholarly disputation; it would have almost certainly dispelled the cheerful atmosphere that had surrounded the reunion of the fellow Paduan students.

'But, tell me,' Hofmann shifted his ground, 'why do you doff the

---

*Harvey never hit upon an adequate solution to this problem, though he 'did look after [the invisible routes] with all possible diligence'. The vessels, which are known today as the capillaries, were first described by Marcello Malpighi (1628–1694), who spied them through a microscope after Harvey's death.

hat of an anatomist, and suddenly put on the hat of an accountant, relying on calculations of how much blood can be transferred from the heart to the arteries in the space of an hour? Such calculations and old wives' tales may have the power to convince the ignorant rabble gathered here today, but true anatomists and natural philosophers require better arguments.'

Despite the efforts of thinkers such as Bacon and Galileo, arithmetic still had no secure place within anatomy or natural philosophy. We recall that at Cambridge University it was classed as a mechanical study for sailors and merchants rather than as a scholarly pursuit. The discipline might reveal something about the *appearance* of things, but nothing of the *causes* that lay behind it, the explanation of which was the true goal of the Aristotelian natural philosopher. An argument based on the quantity of the blood ejected by the heart was therefore invalid and, in Hofmann's phrase, 'the mere trick of an accountant'. As a natural philosopher of the old school, and no innovative Galilean experimenter himself, Harvey felt this criticism keenly.

Hofmann had cleverly manoeuvred Harvey into a corner, from which the choleric Englishman must have restrained a natural urge to come out fighting. 'My frank and very well-wishing friend,' he said, 'as to the precise amount of blood in the body, you may suppose whatever number you wish, but you must agree that it goes around, and in considerable quantity.'

'Be that as it may,' Hofmann brushed the riposte aside, to pursue an even more compelling line of argument, 'it is of little consequence. What I am really anxious to hear is the final cause of your monstrous fiction. For your false invention seems to have no *purpose*. What reason can you give me for the circulation of the blood? You would seem to accuse Nature of superfluity and stupidity! Superfluity, for sending more blood round the body than is necessary for nourishment—something that is utterly contrary to Nature's wisdom, which through attraction draws to an organ no more blood than it requires; and stupidity, for you hold that Nature concocts the blood, distributes it, and then destroys the work it has done, making it impure, only to return it to the heart to be concocted again. In other words, nature concocts in order to concoct? And so on forever? To what *purpose*, I ask again, what is the *cause*? I warn you Harvey, have a care of your philosophic reputation! You impose on Nature the character of an idle artificer, and in doing so you take the Devil's part—for your hypothesis being admitted, what amount of wicked confusion will not follow in all the other works Nature performs?'

Nature was universally believed to be incapable of error. The purification of the blood made sense because nature was transforming a substance from a corrupt into a perfect state, yet for the blood then to become corrupt again, having nourished the body, and to require renewed purification, appeared to suggest that nature was in some way deficient, or in Hofmann's phrase 'capable of folly'. For Harvey to argue this would have been intellectual heresy.

Harvey had no intention of denying nature's perfection, adhering sincerely to the dogma himself, and being conscious of the appalling consequences of challenging it. As an ardent Aristotelian, he also understood only too well Hofmann's demand that he produce a 'final cause' or purpose for his theory. To his dismay, after more than twenty years of investigation and meditation, Harvey had been unable to fathom circulation's final cause—nature's ultimate purpose in designing a circular route for the blood. This must have been acutely embarrassing to him, and he doubtless regarded his theory as philosophically incomplete in consequence. Harvey's anxiety on this overwhelming question may indeed have delayed the penning of his theory by some years. Ultimately, however, while he remained in the dark over the final cause, his specific arguments, philosophical generalizations and the ocular evidence produced by his demonstrations nevertheless convinced him that his thesis ought to be committed to paper. It was a bold and pragmatic decision born of necessity.

In composing his account of the incomplete theory, three choices had lain open to Harvey with regard to the final cause: he could deny its importance and so break faith with Aristotle; he could speculate on it, offering 'likely reasons' for the circulation; or he could ignore the issue altogether. Again with a pragmatism that was exceptional among Aristotelian natural philosophers, Harvey had elected, in the main, to ignore the issue.

This had been a vulnerable position for Harvey to take up, as it had left him open to criticism. Yet he had little choice but to adopt it again now in his duel with Hofmann. 'My dear Hofmann,' he endeavoured to placate the German, 'I admit that I am a very bad philosopher, for I do not know the final cause; I also understand why, in consequence of this, you reject the Circulation. But first you must confess there is a Circulation of the blood, then enquire for what reason it is, for from those things that do happen upon the circulation and the allowance of it, the use and profits accruing can be searched. Then we can search for the final cause; indeed, perhaps you yourself would be good enough to assist me in this endeavour.'

'Pah!' snorted Hofmann, expressing the sort of contempt he usually reserved for his dullest students. 'My dear Hofmann,' Harvey pleaded, 'do not mock.' Yet the German would not be diverted. 'And so Harvey', he announced, 'has admitted it at last—he is a circulator!' By 'circulator' Hofmann meant an empiric who peddled potions at country fairs—the implication being that his arguments were based on experience rather than theory. It was a clever double entendre that the audience would have appreciated.

Harvey took umbrage at anyone who 'tried to make a laughing stock' of him or his theory, but on this occasion he managed to muster up the little patience that remained to him, once more attempting to persuade his old friend that he was 'not mentally deranged'. 'Listen,' he entreated the German, 'you either do not pay attention to me, or fail to grasp my meaning.' Nothing Harvey said, however, could overcome Hofmann's obduracy, and finally the Englishman snapped. Breaking off mid-sentence, Harvey picked up one of the knives from the dissection table and threw it on the floor, before turning away from his old friend and pacing out of the theatre.

Two days after the Altdorf demonstration, Harvey returned to the fray, delivering to Hofmann what he referred to as an epistolary 'hammering'. Reluctant, perhaps, to break a venerable intellectual fellowship, he nevertheless signed off his long letter with expressions of 'goodwill'. Having done so, Harvey rejoined the English diplomatic mission which journeyed from Germany to Prague, where they visited Ketschin Castle, the imposing stronghold of the king of Bohemia and former residence of Rudolph II of Austria. There, a little-known episode took place, which deserves to be told as part of Harvey's story.

Rudolph II was one of the great collectors and patrons of the age, numbering among his courtiers artists such as Paolo Veronese, and masters of the occult sciences including Elizabeth I's astronomer John Dee. In his citadel, the reclusive Rudolph surrounded himself with works of art and the largest collection of curios and rarities in Europe.

The English delegation was permitted to wander through the castle's extensive corridors and apartments, magnificently furnished by Rudolph with mosaics, bronze statues, astronomical instruments, gorgeous paintings and chests overflowing with lavishly bound books. They were especially charmed by the Schant Room, a labyrinthine chamber made up of a series of tiny rooms, housing cupboards filled with Rudolph's cornucopia of exotic collections. In the first small room, one cabinet contained numerous pieces of the finest porcelain, another a yard-long unicorn's horn.

In the very centre of the room, the company was brought to a halt by a collection of clocks of all kinds. There was a clock 'surrounded by a metal ball running around in a grove; from it hung two cords which, when pulled, caused sweet music to sound, though we could not discern whence it came'. Perhaps the most impressive device was in the form of a globe and the heavens. It consisted of a clock with a representation of the celestial and terrestrial spheres, set in motion by various trains and by wheels upon which the earth and the sun and moon revolved, tracing a perfectly circular movement. 'Against the background of gold on the clock's face, coloured green to resemble a field, a buck ran in and out while pursuing hounds gave tongue; in the lower section of the clock, quaint figures danced and music sounded.'

Before Harvey's alert and eager eyes, the human race and the natural world kept mechanical time, as the great globe itself and its brave overhanging firmament revolved by clockwork. In the imagination we may search the Englishman's small, round face, for evidence of interest. He was famous among his diplomatic colleagues for his unquenchable desire to 'satisfy his curiosity' in all intellectual matters, so we may safely assume his attention, and indeed his fascination. We scrutinize his face too, for any trace of recognition, or intuition, that a revolution was about to take place in the world of natural philosophy—a revolution which his ideas helped to bring about.

∽৪ Essay 8 ৪∾

Descartes' clockwork universe

THE FRENCH PHILOSOPHER René Descartes (1596–1650) was fascinated by mechanical clocks. Trained as a lawyer at the University of Poitiers, Descartes had shut up his law books in youth in order to focus on knowledge derived exclusively from either his own mind or from the 'the great book of the world'.

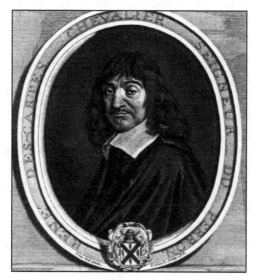

Seventeenth-century engraving of Descartes. A profound loathing for the intricacies of Aristotelian logic, and a series of visionary dreams, convinced Descartes that it was his vocation to renovate natural philosophy.

Descartes' twenties and thirties were spent, in his words, 'travelling, visiting courts, gathering various experiences' and at all times reflecting upon whatever crossed his path. Over the course of his travels, the Frenchman encountered a number of mechanical clocks and saw in them a revolutionary image of humanity, nature and the universe. 'We see that clocks', he wrote in his *Discourse on Method* (1637), published a few months after Harvey's visit to Ketschin, 'have been built by men, but do not for this reason lack the power to move by themselves'. Could the universe, Descartes speculated, have been devised by a sort of 'industrious watch-maker' deity? Could it be 'similar to a clock' rather than to that 'divine animated being' imagined by natural philosophers down the centuries? That is, might not the world be bereft of spirits and invisible forces and run 'mechanically, or automatically, like the actions and motions of a clock'?

If that were the case, Descartes wondered, then might not the body of man also be a machine, similar to the 'many different automata or moving machines the industry of man can devise'? And might not the heart, the central organ of man, also function like a clock, whose mechanical movements follow from the arrangements of its wheels and parts?

Descartes was one of the first natural philosophers to champion Harvey's circulation theory in print. In praising the theory in his *Discourse*, the Frenchman modified it considerably, replacing Harvey's forceful systole with an active diastole, during which the heat of the heart first expands and then expels the blood. Descartes' mind instinctively moved and expressed itself in metaphors drawn from the mechanical world. He compared the heart to a combustion engine driven by a series of explosions occurring at regular intervals, as though by clockwork; he claimed that it also worked (as Harvey had hinted) as a sort of hydraulic pump. 'One may well liken', he wrote, 'the nerves of the animal machine to the pipes of the machines of fountains . . . its animal spirits, of which the heart is the source, to the water that moves these engines.' What was implied and incidental in Harvey became, in Descartes' writings, explicit and central.

The body functioned like a complex machine, Descartes argued, by virtue of the hydraulic system whose centre was the heart, the organ being the source of all bodily heat and motion. Harvey had undermined faith in the idea of the innate pulse-making force of the arteries, and in the belief that the organs attract blood to themselves—the heart alone was responsible for the pulse and the movement of blood. Descartes adapted this idea, arguing that the heart beat automatically, being completely independent of the mind and the soul. The heart was the centre of Descartes' new mechanical philosophy; the vast intellectual superstructure he had constructed stood or fell, the Frenchman declared, on his Harvey-inspired understanding of the heart.

Descartes believed that it was only through deductive, a priori reasoning, rather than the evidence of the senses, that man could arrive at the eternal metaphysical truths. Yet, at the same time, any attempt to understand the natural world ought, he argued, to be based on sensory experience. While Descartes' natural philosophy is clearly based on deductive principles, he nevertheless embraced and promoted a broadly empirical approach to research that is reminiscent at times of the programmes of Bacon and Galileo.

The aim of Descartes' natural philosophy was to identify the mechanical laws governing both the macrocosm and the microcosm. 'There are no rules in mechanics', he declared, 'which do not hold good in physics . . . it is not less natural for a clock, made of the requisite number of wheels, to indicate the hours, than for a tree which has sprung from this or that seed, to produce a particular fruit.' A close observation of a natural phenomenon—a precise measurement of its size, shape and motion—was, Descartes announced, the only sure way of investigating those laws. In the context of the heart, this meant measuring its movements, computing the amount of blood entering and leaving it at every beat. In Descartes' view, an accurate estimate of that figure was no mere 'trick of an accountant'; it was a significant fact which shed light on the mechanical laws determining the organ's motions. Harvey had underrated the importance of his calculation, producing only a very approximate figure; Descartes and his followers tried to establish the exact quantity.

Descartes' writings were intended as an elaborate and extended elegy on Aristotle. The Frenchman declared that there were no phenomena in the universe that could not be explained by 'purely physical causes'—independent of 'mind and thought', as well as an Aristotelian 'final cause'. In elucidating this idea, Descartes again turned to the example of a mechanical clock. When we gaze at a clock, he wrote, we only discern the *effects* of its inner workings—we see the hands moving around the dial, but cannot perceive the reasons for this effect. Such effects are *facts*, which can be observed and agreed upon by qualified philosophers; the reasons for those facts are *causes*, which 'it is impossible to define with any certainty'.

As it was with the clock, so it was with the clockwork universe. 'God works' within it, according to Descartes, 'in an infinity of ways, without it being possible for the mind of man to be aware of which of these means He has chosen to employ . . . [we] shall have done enough if the causes listed are such that the effects they may produce are similar to those we see in the world.' As an illustration of his meaning, Descartes offered the valves of the heart. The result of the action of the valves was to regulate the flow of the blood in one direction, but it would be wrong to think of this consequence as a divine or Aristotelian 'purpose'; it was enough to define it as a mechanical action, and leave it at that.

In discussing 'final causes' Descartes at times sounded like the Harvey who had asked Caspar Hofmann to 'first confess there is a Circulation of the blood, then enquire for what reason it is'. Yet where Harvey's inability to fathom a final cause troubled him deeply, Descartes found in it a reason for celebration. So far as the Frenchman was concerned, Harvey's inability to explain the final cause was immaterial—it was enough to have demonstrated the facts (that is, the effects), which established the circulation.

Descartes' writings ushered in a new intellectual horizon. There would be no place in it for either Galen's vitalism (the idea that the body depended on spirits, and was comprised of organs that were intelligent and alive), Aristotelian causes and first principles, or for the notion that nature did nothing in vain. Descartes' mechanical philosophy (along with the programme of empirical inductive enquiry adumbrated by Bacon) would come to dominate natural philosophy. By 1665 Robert Boyle, the most pre-eminent English natural philosopher of his generation, would refer to the human body as a 'hydraulical engine . . . fram'd and contriv'd by nature', and he compared Nature to 'a great piece of clock-work'. This Cartesian metaphor was prompted by a visit Boyle paid to Strasbourg Cathedral. He had marvelled at the vast clock there which displayed the mechanical circular movements of the sun and moon, and was adorned with moving animal and human figures.

14. Civil War years (the 1640s): 'Anabaptists, fanatics, robbers, and murderers'

THE MOST VOCIFEROUS champions of the circulation theory hailed from the fresh generation of anatomy students nurtured by Descartes' ideas. It was only with the advent of the new mechanical intellectual horizon from the 1640s onwards that Harvey's revolutionary concept came to be fully understood and accepted by natural philosophers. The Englishman's arguments thereafter seemed to carry greater weight, and many of the traditional objections to the theory lost their force. The new generation of young anatomists, who often invoked Harvey as their exemplar and inspiration, investigated the body as though it were an elaborate machine, explicitly rejecting vitalist and Aristotelian principles.

It was the enthusiasm and growing influence of the anatomical vanguard, along with the broader cultural appeal of Harvey's ideas, that ensured the success of the circulation theory. 'With much adoe at last', as one contemporary remarked, 'in about 20 or 30 years [i.e. c.1650]', the theory 'was received in all the Universities in the world'. Harvey's genius finally received recognition, and he became renowned as 'the only man, perhaps, that ever lived to see his owne Doctrine established in his life-time'.

Yet many of the intellectual developments of these years made Harvey uneasy and, during the 1640s, he was compelled to pick up his pen. 'This lower world', he scribbled, in a hand that had deteriorated further with the onset of old age, 'is so continuous with the superior realms, that all its motions and changes seem to take their origin from thence and be governed by them.' Perhaps with Descartes in mind, Harvey used a mechanical clock to illustrate this statement, along with the corollary notion, that spiritual forces animate the world, suffusing even artificial devices. 'Scarcely any elemental body', he mused, 'does not in its actions surpass its own powers . . . when our clocks do faithfully tell all the hours of the day and of the night,—do these not seem to partake of another body besides the elements, and of a body more divine? If by the dominion and rule of Art such excellent works are daily produced as do surpass the powers of the materials themselves, what then shall we think can be done by the precept and rule of Nature [which has been fashioned by] the hand of God?'

Harvey's words were part of his vast treatise on the subject of generation (i.e. the propagation of living organisms), published as *De Generatione Animalium* in 1651 and translated in 1653 as *Anatomical Exercitations, Concerning the Generation of Living Creatures*. It was Descartes, as well as Aristotle and Fabricius (both of whom had written on the same theme), who called the Kentishman back to his writing table. Gratified as he was by his growing celebrity, and the increasing appeal of his circulation theory, Harvey despised the mechanical philosophy that had facilitated its success.

When he turned to the heart and the blood in animals in his new book, Harvey was at pains to distinguish his views from those of Descartes. The Frenchman had, he declared, not only misinterpreted the movements of the heart (arguing for an active diastole), but also the cause of its motion. The heart moved, Harvey averred, of its own accord, because of the 'pulsative faculty' or 'power of soul' within it. The organ was 'an autonomous living thing' rather than a clock or a mechanical pump—as Descartes claimed, and as he himself had previously implied.

The heart, Harvey went on, regenerated the 'vital heat' of the blood, which was also enlivened by an inherent 'vital motion'. The liquid was full of 'spirits' too, which 'move the whole mechanism of the body as they flow continuously from the arteries'. Because of this, blood could be described as:

> the immediate instrument of the soul and its first abode . . . as it seems to participate in some other more divine body and is perfused with divine animal heat it is analogous to the element of the stars. In so far as it is spirit, it is the hearth, the goddess Vesta, the household deity, innate heat, the sun of the microcosm, Plato's fire . . . it preserves and nourishes itself and grows by its wavering and perpetual motion. It also deserves the name of spirit as it dispenses [radical moisture] to all the rest the same substance . . . [just as] the Sun and the Moon impart life to the earth.

Sensing perhaps that such philosophical-poetical epiphanies had, in a world enthralled by Descartian and Baconian ideas, lost some of their power to convince, Harvey confronted the mechanical philosophers head-on. In 'assigning only a material cause', he thundered, and 'deducing the cause of natural things from an involuntary and causal occurrence of the elements [they] do not reach that which is chiefly concerned in the operations of nature . . . namely the divine agent, and God in nature, whose operations are guided with the highest artifice, providence, and wisdom, and do all tend to some certain end, and are all produced for some certain good'.

Yet it was too late for such arguments. When Harvey came to the end of his gargantuan manuscript, we may imagine him putting down his pen more in sorrow than in anger, realizing that he could do little to stop the mechanical-empirical revolution. Descartes' philosophy made redundant so much of what Harvey valued in natural philosophy, including the very principles that had inspired his circulation theory. Harvey's theory had, against the author's wishes, helped usher in the new dispensation, yet under that dispensation it could never have been born.

The concept of the body politic had, as we have seen, influenced Harvey's thinking on the heart. In dedicating *De motu cordis* to Charles I, Harvey had explicitly promoted the idea that the king was as supremely necessary to society as the heart was to the body, or the sun to the universe.

Charles, who famously believed that 'Kings are not bound to give an account of their actions but to God alone', must have been gratified to be hailed as England's sun-heart-king. Intellectual support was most welcome to a ruler who often felt beleaguered, especially by Parliament, which he had summarily dismissed in 1629. In 1640, after an eleven-year hiatus, Charles took the humiliating step of recalling Parliament in order to entreat the House to levy a tax on his people. Like his father before him, Charles' greatest problem was financing his court and military campaigns, in a period of high inflation. In presenting his case for a national tax at Westminster, the king argued that if he imposed on his subjects, it was only because he wished to spend the money on their improvement. Taxes, he declared, were like 'vapours rising out of the earth, gathered into a cloud'; the cloud, in turn, raining down 'sweet refreshing showers on the same fields from which they had been first exhaled.' Charles' use of this Harveian–Aristotelian metaphor suggests that he may indeed have followed Harvey's advice to read *De motu cordis* 'at the same time contemplat[ing] the Principle of Man's Body, and the Image of your Kingly power'.

The 1640 Parliament was unresponsive. They would not further the King's cause until Charles renounced his claim to be 'a sovereign power . . . above the laws and statutes of this kingdom'; the Protestant faith was also to be confirmed as the 'birthright and inheritance' of the English people. The autocratic Charles, whom many suspected of Catholic tendencies, was widely regarded as a threat to the inalienable political and religious rights of all Englishmen.

An uneasy stalemate followed, but conflict erupted again in 1642, this time in the form of full-scale civil war. The parliamentary forces, known as the Roundheads, marched against the monarch under Oliver Cromwell's banner, while the Royalist Cavaliers rallied around their king. Harvey had no doubt where his allegiance lay, describing the Roundheads as a pack of 'Anabaptists, fanatics, robbers, and murderers.'

Harvey proved his steadfastness by staying close to his king, even on the field of battle. During the bloody skirmish at Edgehill in 1642, the king's two sons were committed to Harvey's care. Harvey told a friend that he 'withdrew with them under a hedge, and tooke out of his pocket a booke and read; but he had not read very long before a Bullet of a great Gun grazed on the ground near him, which made him remove his station'. We may recall here the popular belief that the kings of England, and other royal persons, were always 'wont to remain among' their yeomen during battles, 'the Prince showing by this where his chief strength did consist'.

Yet even the loyalty of men such as Harvey could not save the king against the tenacity of his enemies. After six years of war, the Royalists were finally defeated, and the republican Commonwealth was founded. In 1649, Charles was beheaded in front of the Banqueting House at Whitehall, the English thereby becoming the first modern people to cut off the head of their king on a constitutional principle.

De motu cordis was a species of Royalist anatomy. Yet despite Harvey's overt political aims, his book unwittingly encouraged radical ideas with regard to the body politic, just as it did in the world of natural philosophy. In entering the culture and the language Harvey's circulation theory generated waves of change over which he had no control. In arguing that the same blood nourished every part of the body (against Galen's idea of two distinct blood types) Harvey appeared to some to undermine the hierarchy of both the blood and the organs. It was appalling, conservative critics argued, to imagine that the nobler organs, such as the lungs, could be sustained by the same blood as the inferior organs—why, it would be like offering the king the same dish as a country bumpkin, a contradiction of the laws of nature, which were the laws of God.

Harvey's suggestion that the heart worked like a set of water bellows or a pump proved to be even more dangerous, especially after Descartes adopted the idea. If the heart was indeed a pump then the most appropriate parallel for the organ would no longer be a king, but a sort of steward who performed his office diligently, consistently and mechanically, without thinking. Better still, Cromwell's supporters reckoned, the heart might be compared to Parliament.

The political theorist James Harrington dexterously turned Harvey's ideas to radical ends, fashioning from them a variety of republican political-anatomy. Parliament, he claimed, in a book dedicated to Cromwell, was the true 'heart' of the body politic. 'Consisting of two ventricles [i.e. the Commons and the Lords], the one greater and replenished with a grosser store, the other less and full of a purer', the heart 'sucketh in and gusheth forth the life blood' of the Commonwealth, so sustaining it in 'a perpetual circulation'. Historical events bore Harrington out, for how could the heart be the king, or the king the heart, when the body politic survived Charles' execution in 1649?

As the Cartesian dispensation extended its hegemony across Europe, the concept of the body politic gradually lost relevance. The heart was now regarded as an engine or a pump at the centre of a microcosmic machine; a machine was an artificial device, which could not possibly be organized according to an organic hierarchy. This idea was eloquently set forth in *Leviathan* (1651), Thomas Hobbes' masterpiece of political philosophy.

An acquaintance of Harvey, Hobbes celebrated the theory of the circulation of the blood in the opening pages of *Leviathan*. The political philosopher's understanding of his friend's theory was, however, filtered through his reading of Descartes. He described the Harveian heart as 'a great piece of machinery in which one wheel gives motion to another'. Harvey's discovery had, Hobbes argued, revealed that the body functioned like an artificial device, a truth that could be applied to the body politic. Society might be described as a mechanical body formed by social contract, a machine assembled rationally by man. Hobbes declared monarchy to be the best form of government but only because it was the most perfect artificial state, not because it had been ordained by God, or nature; a monarch, he said, also had a duty to honour the 'contract' he had signed with his people. Staunch Royalists such as Harvey were appalled by key aspects of the argument, as well as by the mechanical premise on which it was based.

The body politic was only one of countless correspondences between the microcosm and the macrocosm that became redundant under the new mechanical dispensation. If the body were a machine, then searching for parallels between it and the world of nature (or the celestial world) was pointless. The various parts of the mechanical body were to be measured and weighed, not linked with other entities in the chain of being; knowledge now focused on quantification rather than on the identification of correspondences—a fanciful and superfluous activity which could be left entirely to the poets. Poets and natural philosophers now ceased to be intellectual brothers—the heirs of John Donne and William Harvey would no longer share a common language.

Descartes' philosophy left no room for what he called 'occult forces in stones or plants . . . amazing and marvellous sympathies'; consequently, it had no place for metaphors either. On this point the Frenchman was at one with Bacon, who wrote that 'all ornaments of speech . . . similitudes, treasury of eloquence, and such like emptinesses [should] be utterly dismissed'. If nature was comprised of 'things singular and unmatched' why should language and the mind devise 'for them conjugates and parallels and relatives that do not exist'? Partly in consequence of Bacon and Descartes' influence, around the middle of the seventeenth century, 'all deductions from Metaphors, Parables, Allegories', as the great prose stylist and physician Sir Thomas Browne put it, became bereft of 'force'; thereafter, only 'real and rigid interpretations' had the power to convince.

Thomas Sprat, historian and member of the Royal Society (which would receive its charter in 1662), issued an *ex cathedra* decree regarding new stylistic standards for works of natural philosophy. Authors were to deliver 'so many *things* in an equal number of *words*', to render their words as unambiguous as 'numbers', using them as transparent tokens that revealed objects *as they really are*. Only in this way could men avoid confusion and discord, which had been so evident of late in politics as well as natural philosophy. A clear, accurate and impartial description of facts, a perspicuous description of the measurements of a phenomenon, and the laws governing its motion, were now all that was required. The natural philosopher must, he implied, become invisible—a dispassionate observer of natural phenomena—and the reader a virtual witness of his experiments.

Harvey's comparisons of the heart to a set of water bellows and to a sort of pump were, in a sense, the analogies to end all analogies. Hit upon perhaps in a moment of exuberant fancy, expressed without careful consideration of potential philosophical and political consequences, and certainly not regarded by Harvey as any more significant than the myriad natural metaphors he employed throughout his oeuvre, the parallel heralded the beginning of a new intellectual era. Descartes latched on to it, and made it the cornerstone of his vision of the body, and of a philosophy in which analogies would lose all their capacity to persuade and beguile.

With the arrival of Descartes' philosophy, the heart also lost much of its fascination. In becoming an insentient pump at the centre of a purely material and mechanical body, it no longer offered a home to thoughts, a nursery to the imagination, or a citadel to the soul. For the Frenchman, the brain was where intellectual action began and developed. Man was distinguished from automaton animals (who were all body) by virtue of the reasoning power of his brain; henceforth man's identity, as an individual as well as a species, would be forged there—'I think,' Cartesian man declared, 'therefore I am.'

The brain also became the official residence of the soul, which Descartes located at the organ's centre in the pineal gland. Mind and soul were rendered virtually synonymous; the intimate ties between both the body and the mind, and between the soul and the body, were cut; the physiological was divorced from the psychological. It became preposterous, in this new mechanical universe, to suppose that the body could think or that a man's personality might be determined by the four humours.

15. Last years (the 1650s):
'Shitt-breeches'

DURING THE CIVIL WAR, Harvey lost numerous possessions, and all of his research papers, when the Roundheads ransacked his London lodgings. 'Of all the losses he sustained, no grief', according to a friend, 'was so crucifying to him as the loss of his papers, which for love or money he could never retrieve or obtain.' These documents contained details of Harvey's countless experiments on animals, as well perhaps as various draft treatises which he had hoped to publish.

Under the English Republic Harvey was classified as a 'delinquent' because of his close association with the executed king. He was banished, at the beginning of the 1650s, 'to a distance of not less than twenty miles from London on pain of imprisonment'. Harvey was probably assessed for various forced loans by Parliament too, and compelled to hand over thousands of pounds. It was around this troubled time that Elizabeth Harvey died; Harvey mourned the loss of the woman who had been his 'dear loving' wife for more than forty years. Harvey also lost three of his brothers, perhaps as casualties of the political conflict or its aftermath. With their death, the close-knit Harvey fellowship was dissolved.

The private medical practice of the political exile was greatly diminished, as many of his patients had been prominent members of Charles' court. In any case, Harvey displayed little enthusiasm now for medical work. When approached for advice or treatment, he would decline to help all but 'special friends'.

When the republic eventually relaxed restrictions on Harvey's movements, the widower elected to live a retired life with his brother Eliab in Bishopsgate, London. His days in Cockaine House, Broad Street, were passed in great physical discomfort. A martyr to the gout, friends remembered how Harvey would seek relief by sitting with his legs in a bucket of freezing water, on the roof of the house, 'till he was almost dead with cold'. Then he would suddenly get up and 'betake himself to the stove' to warm them.

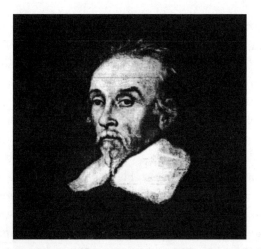

Harvey in the 1650s. Afflictions have visibly diminished him into Shakespeare's emblem of the penultimate 'age of man'—the 'lean and slippered pantaloon', as though the yellow bile in his body has turned black, the choler into melancholy.

In 1652 Harvey's sufferings became increasingly acute until one day (or so a friend's story went) he sent for a physician friend. 'Acquainting him with his intention to die by laudanum that night', Harvey 'desired he would come next morning to take care of his papers and affairs.' Yet if Harvey did indeed swallow the opium, the dose proved insufficient to kill him.

As Harvey crawled painfully towards death there were some consolations. He took up the habit of drinking coffee, brewed in a special 'Coffey pot', thereby becoming famed as one of very first Englishmen 'wont to drinke' the 'blacke as soot' beverage. Physicians believed that the drink comforted the heart, aided digestion, alleviated the gout and fortified one against lethargy of the brain.

Harvey's weakening heart is also rumoured to have drawn comfort and stimulation from a 'pretty young wench' whom he employed 'to wayte on him'. Friends gossiped that he 'made use of' the girl at night 'for warmeth-sake, and tooke care of her in his Will'. In that testament, which was compiled at this time, Harvey acknowledged with an annuity of £20 'the diligence and the service' of one Alice Garth, who may be the woman in question.

The venerable natural philosopher, now in his seventies, derived solace too from the twin gods of his idolatry and ambition—worldly success and intellectual renown. We may recall here that two representations of the goddess Fortune were carved on the Gate of Virtue at Caius College, Cambridge—one goddess holding a bag of gold, the other a palm and a laurel wreath. These sculptures symbolized the college founder's belief that it was only through wisdom, 'and learning grafted in grace and virtue' that men come to wealth and immortality.

Harvey was living testimony to the truth of this motto. Having dedicated his life to intellectual labour, he now reaped the rewards. Despite the best efforts of Parliament, the yeoman's son, and unrepentant Royalist, clung tenaciously to his personal fortune of around £20,000. Part of this money he bequeathed to the College of Physicians, so that it could build a library and a museum at Amen Corner, to be named after him.

That noble building, done in the grandiose style of rustic Roman architecture Harvey favoured, was completed in early 1653. A white marble statue of Harvey, attired in his doctoral robes, greeted visitors at the entrance. An inscription beneath the figure proudly informed them that the benefactor of the buildings was the eldest son of Thomas Harvey of Folkestone.

At the official opening Harvey was elected president of the college. The 'munificent old man' an eyewitness reported, 'gave thanks for the dignity', which was tantamount, he said, to being elected 'prince of all the doctors in England'—a dangerous yet characteristic monarchical allusion. Harvey regretted, however, that he must ask 'to be excused from the office' on the grounds of 'infirmity and age'.

Through his association with the college, and its magnificent buildings, Harvey hoped that his name would live on beyond his death, as a sort of second Thomas Linacre. In his will Harvey left the college some of the many lands he had acquired, with the instruction that the rent accrued from them fund an annual banquet. During the yearly feast a Latin oration was, he stipulated, to be delivered, commemorating all the benefactors of the college (himself included), and containing an exhortation to fellows to diligently study the mysteries of nature. Harvey also left to the college some books and papers from his library, in the hope that this would ensure their survival.*

Yet Harvey must have known that *De motus cordis* would be his true monument—the 'son', as one admirer described it, which the 'childless doctor' bequeathed to future generations. Writing to a fellow author Harvey had expressed the hope that his friend's 'little anatomical book' would 'live for ever and tell the glory of your name to posterity long after even marble has perished'. He surely harboured similar ambitions for his own volume. 'Perish my thoughts', he would tell friends, 'if they are empty and . . . wrong . . . let my writings lie neglected. [However] if I am right, sometime, in the end, the human race will not disdain the truth.'

* It did not. These items would be lost to the flames of the Great Fire of 1666, along with the college buildings and the statue of Harvey at Amen Corner.

If ever Harvey expressed doubts about his posthumous fame, the numerous disciples who gathered around him in his twilight years would try to set his mind at ease. Sitting beside the grand old man '2 or 3 hours together in his meditating apartment discoursing', these young men would remind him of the 'tireless industry in the advancement of natural philosophy' that had made him 'the chiefest glory and ornament' of both the College of Physicians and of his country.

Basking in the glow of their praise, Harvey would rouse himself momentarily to speak again with 'admirable readiness' and a 'cheerful countenance' of the work that had been the ruling passion of his life. Yet invariably he would soon lapse back into melancholy. How could he be happy? he asked his acolytes, employing his favourite body-politic metaphor, 'when the Commonwealth is full of intestine troubles, and I myself as yet upon the high seas'. Even the memory of his circulation theory was often as wormwood to him. 'Much better', he would reflect, 'is it oftentimes to grow wise at home and in private, than by publishing what you have amassed with infinite labour, to stir up tempests that may rob you of your peace and quiet for the rest of your days.'

Harvey's theory had indeed stirred up a tempest in the world of anatomy, and provoked discord among the physicians, many of whom feared that it would revolutionize medicine.* It also produced powerful philosophical and cultural vibrations. Having grown out of the prevailing culture and language of the time, it in turn exercised a profound influence on them. The theory encouraged radical ideas with regard to the body politic. Indeed, it was not without justice that in 1653 a poet addressed Harvey as the 'disturber of

---

*Their fears proved to be unfounded. After the publication of *De motu cordis*, most physicians (Harvey included) continued to use therapies such as bloodletting, as though the blood moved within the body in accordance with Galen's theories, rather than in a rapid circle. Bloodletting in fact survived as a common treatment well into the eighteenth century. And while the circulation theory inspired one or two new medical treatments, such as blood transfusions, these were dismissed as worthless by most physicians and by Harvey himself.

the quiet of Physicians! [The] seditious Citizen of the Physical Common Wealth! Who first of all durst oppose an opinion confirm'd for so many ages by the consent of all.' One wonders whether Harvey read these words and reflected on the role his theories may have indirectly played in the downfall of his king. In one version of the body politic, yeomen are assigned the role of the ribs, for they were regarded as 'the king's citadel, constructed so that the heart, might be protected like a king'; looking back, did Harvey consider that, in promoting his radical theory, he had unwittingly done his sovereign less than 'yeoman's service'?

Harvey had also unintentionally lent inspiration, and credence, to Descartes' profoundly influential mechanical philosophy. The ailing anatomist was now celebrated as the great English prophet of Descartes' clockwork universe. Through his explorations of the body's interior, the poet Martin Lluelyn wrote, Harvey had unveiled mechanical workings that had been hidden to previous ages:

> There thy *Observing* Eye first found the Art
> Of all the *Wheels* and *Clock-work* of the *Heart* . . .
> What secret Engines tune the *Pulse*, whose din
> By *Chimes without, Strikes* how things fare *within*.

The long shadow of Descartes was often cast over Harvey's conversations with his disciples, many of whom subscribed to the new philosophy, much to their mentor's annoyance. When one acolyte asked him which philosophical books he ought to read, Harvey bid his pupil 'goe to the Fountain head, and read Aristotle . . . and [he] did call the Neoteriques [i.e. the new theorists of the mechanical philosophy] *shitt-breeches*'.

In the early summer of 1657, with Cromwell ruling over the Commonwealth as Lord Protector, the seventy-nine-year-old

William Harvey suffered a serious stroke. Apparently, he once again discussed suicide with his friends, but he began to sink so fast that such a step was deemed unnecessary. On the morning of 3 June at about ten o'clock, Harvey tried to speak but 'found he had the dead palsey in his tongue'. Realizing what was to become of him he sent for his brother Eliab and his young nephews. When they had come up to him, Harvey mustered the strength to present to one of his brother's sons 'the minute watch with which he had made his experiments', as a 'remembrance of him'. Harvey then made a gesture to his apothecary 'to let him blood in the tongue, which did little or no good . . . so he ended his dayes'.

And so William Harvey—dutiful son of the yeoman Thomas Harvey, and author of one of the most magnificent generalizations in what we now call the 'history of science'—humbly rendered, to quote his will, his 'soul to Him that gave it'. It is fitting that his final moments should have featured both a watch—the symbol of the new mechanical epoch that had just begun—and an ineffectual attempt at bloodletting—the emblem of a Galenic age that was passing. Few men deserve to be regarded as the mainspring of that vast historical change more than William Harvey.

Acknowledgements

I WOULD LIKE TO thank the staff of the various libraries in which I carried out my research: the Bodleian Library (especially the staff of the Upper Reading Room), the Wellcome Unit for the History of Medicine Library, the Radcliffe Science Library, and the History Faculty Library (all of which are libraries of Oxford University); the British Library (particularly the staff at Science 2); the London Library; and the public library at Botley, which, at the time of writing, thankfully remains open.

I would like to give my special thanks to James Cox, College Archivist, Gonville and Caius College, Cambridge, for kindly showing me all college documents relating to Harvey; and to the student guides of Padua University who gave me a guided tour of 'il Bo', and its magnificent anatomy theatre.

I am enormously grateful to my editors at Chatto & Windus, Penelope Hoare and Parisa Ebrahimi, whose comments on the early drafts of this book have been invaluable. The book has also benefited from the editorial expertise and intellectual agility of Anna Wright, my ideal reader. Thanks also to Clara Farmer, for her help in coming up with the title.

The help of my former agent, Camilla Hornby, in developing the idea for this book, and in drafting the proposal, was crucial.

Without her expertise and enthusiasm this book would not exist. The encouragement and advice of my current agent, Karolina Sutton, has helped me enormously in taking the project through to its end. My thanks to them both.

I would like to express my appreciation for Chiara Raso, Gabriella Raso and Bianca Brilla, of the T.T.S. Aosta school of languages, who helped with the translations from Latin and Italian; Dr Caroline Barnes, who, as always, gave me some excellent suggestions; and Annamaria Biavasco, who explored Padua with me, and offered me comments and inspiration. Thanks also to the following people for their advice, help and support: Beppe Narizzano, Sinead Garrigan-Mattar, Jamie Glazebrook, Tracey Carroll, Mary Fanning, Paul and Anne-Marie Wright, Lol Reynolds (1926–2010), Frances Mary Wright (1920–2003), Giles Gordon (1940–2003), and Mark Slater.

Notes

Prologue

As no verbatim record has survived for Harvey's Altdorf lecture my reconstruction is based on the following sources: Harvey (1928; 1961) and especially Harvey's "Letter to Caspar Hofmann," dated 20 May 1636, published in Harvey (1990). I have also drawn on descriptions of contemporary vivisections, such as Hesler's (1959). Secondary sources consulted include French (1994) and Whitteridge (1971). My description of Harvey's appearance is derived from Aubrey (1972). My account of the English diplomatic mission comes from Springell (1963).

Chapter 1

For biographical facts I have relied (here, and throughout my book) on Keynes' comprehensive life of Harvey (1966), and to a much lesser extent on Chauvois (1961), Keele (1965), and Power (1897).

For my outline of Harvey's family background, and for the descriptions of Kent, I have drawn on Fuller (1662). For the social context I have relied on useful recent studies of the period by Pritchard (1999) and Thomas (2009), which are the sources for most of the quotations in this chapter. Campbell (1942) is the classic study of the status and characteristics of English yeomen in this period and it is the basis of my comments on the subject here.

My sketch of Harvey's personality is drawn from the letters of the Earl of Arundel and Harvey's father-in-law, Lancelot Browne, which are reproduced in Springell (1963) and Keynes (1966). Harvey's descriptions of nature are taken from Harvey (1653; 1961), and his cider recipe from Keynes (1966).

Chapter 2

For my account of Caius College and student life at Cambridge I have relied heavily on Brooke (1985) and Morgan & Brooke (2004). I have also consulted Venn (1901), Pritchard (1999) and the contemporary documents "Letter from Queen Elizabeth" (1838) and *Statutes of Queen Elizabeth* (1838).

Kearney (1970) and Cressy (1970) were useful for my account of the social composition of the college. The references to Marlowe are taken from Nicholl (1992). Harvey's decision to "embrace medicine" was reported by his friend Charles Scarburgh (see Payne [1957]).

Chapter 3

In addition to the sources mentioned in my notes to chapter 2, I have drawn, for my description of Harvey's studies, on Costello (1958), Feingold (1984), French (1994), Whitteridge (1971), Matsen (1977), and Schmitt (1983). My account of Harvey's Classical studies relies on Fraser-Harris (1934). The description of the state of medical education at Cambridge draws on Allen (1946).

For my description of Caius library and the works it contained I have referred to *List* (1850), and James (1907). Information on Harvey's copy of Galen's *Miscellaneous Writings* can be found in Harvey (1907). All quotations relating directly to Harvey's attitudes and activities at Cambridge come from Scarburgh (Payne [1957]).

Essay 1

For my account of the history of anatomy before Harvey I have used: French (1979; 1999; 2000), Lind (1975), Singer (1957), and Wear et al.

(1985). For my description of Vesalius I have, in addition to these sources, drawn on Vesalius (1949), Hesler (1959), and O'Malley (1964). References to Harvey's choleric character come from Aubrey (1972).

Chapter 4

My account of Harvey's experiences at Dover is taken from Aubrey (1972); Harvey's angry exclamations appear in some of his letters (dating from a later period) published in Harvey (1935). My description of Harvey's decision to go abroad, and his attitude to travel, is from Scarburgh (Payne [1957]).

The principal source for my evocation of Renaissance Padua is Borgherini (1917). Coryate (1978) and Evelyn (1983) also provided some of the local color. The following accounts of the English contingent at Padua have also been useful: Lytton Sells (1947) and Woolfson (1998). It was Aubrey (1972) who reported Harvey's fondness for fingering and drawing his dagger.

For my account of Harvey's Paduan studies I have relied on French (1994), Whitteridge (1971), Bylebyl (1979b), Matsen (1977), Ongaro et al. (2006), and Evelyn (1983). Harvey's own recollections of his medical studies are from Harvey (1961). Material relating to Aristotle is largely taken from Randall (1940; 1961), and Schmitt (1983).

Essay 2

For the history of the cult of the sacred heart I have consulted Bainvel (1924). Harvey's references to the religious aspects of the heart and the blood come from Harvey (1653; 1961). The preacher quoted at the conclusion of the chapter is John Donne.

Chapter 5

My description of the theatre at Padua draws on Klestinec (2004), Ferrari (1987), Rupp (1990), Sawday (1995), Brockbank (1968), and Underwood (1963).

My sketch of Fabricius, and his ideas, is based on Cole (1944), Cunningham (1985), Fabricius (1933; 1942), Pazzini (1957), Randall (1940; 1961), Wear (1983).

As no verbatim record is available of the anatomical lectures Fabricius gave at Padua University, my dramatized account has been concocted from these sources, along with Bylebyl (1979b), Hesler (1959), French (1999), and Ongaro et al. (2006).

My account of the cadavers used for dissections relies on Park (1994) and Carlino (1999). My evocation of Harvey's examination is based on Harvey's diploma, which is reproduced by Payne (1908).

Chapter 6

The evocations of early seventeenth-century London that appear at various places in this book are based on: Ackroyd (2000), Baron (1997), Picard (2003), Pritchard (1999), Prockter (1979), and Stow (1956).

Keynes (1966) reproduces Harvey's marriage license, Lancelot Browne's letter, and information relating to James I's attempt to levy Harvey. Harvey's description of his wife and her "parrat" appears in Harvey (1653); his opinions on sex are recorded by Aubrey (1972).

My account of the College of Physicians, and Harvey's association with the institution, relies on: Keynes (1966), *Appendix* (1696?), Clark (1964), French (1994), and Whitteridge (1971).

My description of St Bartholomew's Hospital, and Harvey's employment there, draws on Keynes (1966; 1974). Keynes (1966) reproduces Harvey's prescription for the man suffering from rheumatism.

My general comments on medicine and medical treatment in the period are based on Beier (1988), French & Wear (1989), Sloan (1996), Thompson (1928), Traister (2001), Wear (2000), and Wear et al. (1985).

Chapter 7

For the sources of my comments on medicine and medical treatment, see the notes to chapter 6 (above). My account of Harvey's dealings with Sir

Walter Smith is based on primary sources quoted by Keynes (1966), as is my description of James I's medical condition and death, and my evocation of Harvey's conversations with Charles I. Quotations from Harvey's letters are from Harvey (1935).

Harvey's attitude to titles and honors is reported by Scarburgh (Payne [1957]). My comments on the Harvey family and its business dealings are derived from Fuller (1662). For details of Harvey's land and property speculations I have used Harvey Family (2001; 2002). Thomas Harvey's advice to his sons appears in his will.

Chapter 8

I have reconstructed Harvey's lecture from the following sources: his manuscript lecture notes (Harvey [1961; 1964]), his published and unpublished writings (Harvey [1875; 1907; 1928; 1959; 1990]), as well as near contemporary sources (Fabricius [1942], Hesler [1959], and Vesalius [1949]).

I have also used the following secondary sources: French (1979), French (1994), Whitteridge (1971), Power (1897), Keynes (1966), Ferrari (1987), Klestinec (2004), Keele (1965), Payne (2007), and Wilson (1987).

Chapter 9

The details of Harvey's furniture come from his will (Harvey [1990]). The description of Harvey's research chamber relies on Shapin (1988); the evocation of his menagerie is based on Cole (1957), Keynes (1966), and all of Harvey's published and unpublished writings: Harvey (1875; 1907; 1928; 1959; 1961; 1964; 1990).

The anecdote concerning Harvey and the swallows, and that of Harvey scouring the woods, come from Keynes (1966). Harvey himself wrote the account of the dissections he made in the royal parks (Harvey 1653; 1928).

For my account of Harvey's private research program, his published and unpublished writings are, once again, the main source. In addition,

I have relied on French (1994), Whitteridge (1971), and Cunningham (1985). For my description of the specifically Fabrician aspect of Harvey's endeavor, I have drawn on the sources mentioned in my notes on Fabricius' ideas (notes for chapter 5, above). The anecdote of Harvey examining the young man's exposed heart is taken from Harvey (1653).

Essay 3

Comments by Harvey's contemporaries on his vivisections are derived from Keynes (1966) and French (1994). The poem purporting to describe one of Harvey's vivisections can be found in Harvey (1907).

For the history of vivisection prior to Harvey I have used French (1999). For contemporary attitudes to vivisection, I have drawn on French (1994; 1999), Guerrini (1989), Maehle (1993), Maehle & Trohler (1987), and Shrugg (1968).

Chapter 10

For details of the sources I have used in compiling my account of Harvey's private research program, see notes on sources for chapter 9 (above). My description of Harvey's quantitative experiments draws on Jevons (1962); the comments on Harvey's experiments generally were influenced by Banyon (1938). Fabricius (1933) gives an account of his experiments on the veins.

The quotation regarding the birth of the circulation theory is a conflation of Harvey's famous comments to Robert Boyle on the subject (reproduced in Keynes [1966]), and the account that appears in *De motu cordis* (Harvey [1928]). Bates' commentary on Harvey's account was useful (Bates [1992]).

Essay 4

The comparison between Harvey and Bacon was made by Chauvois (1961). All of the biographical and anecdotal material in this essay was supplied by Aubrey (1972).

The quotations from Bacon come from Bacon (1884). I have also drawn on the following sources in my description of his philosophy: Henry (2002), Jardine (1974), and Russell (1946). My comments on Galileo are based on Heilbron (2010).

My account of Harvey's experiments borrows from Banyon (1938), Jevons (1962), French (1994), and Whitteridge (1971). Harvey's remarks on Aristotle, and his quotations from the Greek philosopher, appear in Harvey (1653). Harvey's comments on the circulation theory are from *De motu cordis* (Harvey [1928]).

Chapter 11

Virtually all of the quotations from Harvey are taken from *De motu cordis* AND *De Circulatione Sanguinis* (Harvey [1928]), but I have also occasionally drawn on Harvey (1653; 1961) as well as some of the letters that appear in Harvey (1990). My account of Harvey's demonstrations, and the debate that followed them, also relies on French (1994).

It was Robert Fludd (Keynes [1966]) who described the spectators watching Harvey with "lynx-like eyes." It was Aubrey (1972) who mentioned Harvey's appalling handwriting. My account of the writing of *De motu cordis* is informed by Bylebyl (1973).

Essay 5

For this essay, and the essay that follows, I am heavily indebted to the brilliant pioneer work of Pagel (1951; 1957; 1967; 1976), whose writings patiently and convincingly reconstruct the landscape of Harvey's mental world.

Quotations from Harvey come mostly from *De motu cordis* (Harvey [1928]), but I also draw on other published and unpublished writings (i.e. Harvey 1959; 1961). Quotations from Donne are taken from Donne (1971). Poynter (1960) is the source of my comments on the possible biographical connections between Donne and Harvey.

In describing the concept of the microcosm and the macrocosm I have used Thomas (1971) and Tillyard (1943). My comments on the idea of the body-politic draw on Hale (1971) and LeGoff (1989); those on Harvey's political views are informed by Hill (1964). I have also quoted material relating to these concepts reproduced in Pritchard (1999) and Thomas (2009). It was Aubrey (1972) who recorded Harvey's references to his two meditating chambers.

Essay 6

For my use of the work of Pagel and for my quotations from Harvey and Donne, see notes for Essay 5 (above). The quotations from Robert Fludd are taken from Fludd (1992). My description of Fludd's philosophy, and of alchemical and hermetical studies generally, also draws on Huffman (1988), Debus (1978), Moran (2006), Nicholl (1980), and Webster (1982). For my account of the connections between Harvey and Fludd I have relied on the writings of Debus (1961; 1970).

My discussion of the idea of the perfect circle was inspired by Huntley (1951), Jung (1980), and Nicholson (1950). My comments on the concept of circulation prior to Harvey draw on Bayon (1939) and Young (2003)

Essay 7

For the source of my quotations from Harvey, see notes for Essay 5 (above). For the source of my descriptions of London, see notes to chapter 6 (above), though I should give special mention to Stow (1956), who was my main source for this essay.

My comments on trade and money draw on Valenze (2006). My account of pumps and pumping devices in the period rely on Keele (1965), Whitteridge (1971), French (1994), and Basalla (1962). Aubrey (1972) is (inevitably) the source for everything vivid and anecdotal relating to Harvey.

Chapter 12

The criticisms of Harvey's theory, and of his skill as a physician, are taken from Aubrey (1972), Keynes (1966), and French (1994). The favourable comments appear in French (1994), Bayon (1939) and Pagel (1957; 1967). The quotations from the poets were collected by Young (2003). The long quotation from Fludd was reproduced by Keynes (1966).

Chapter 13

This chapter dramatizes a disputation between Harvey and Hofmann, which may have taken place at Altdorf University. Scholars are divided as to whether a verbal exchange actually occurred in the auditorium, or whether their discussion was confined to the letters they penned soon after their meeting. I favor the view (held for example by Chauvois [1961]) that there was a war of spoken words, which was subsequently continued in writing. Using the letters of the antagonists I have recreated the sort of verbal duel that many commentators believe to have taken place.

My dramatisation is based on modern translations of Caspar Hofmann's letter to Harvey of 19 May 1636, as well as the criticisms of Harvey contained in his book *Responsio ad duas exercitationes Anatomicas postremas G. Harvei etc. De Circulatione sanguinis* (Paris, 1652); both of these are discussed and quoted in Ferrario et al. (1960). My main source for Harvey's statements is his "Letter to Caspar Hofmann," dated 20 May 1636 (Harvey [1990]); I have also drawn on Harvey (1928). The works of Pagel (1951) and French (1994) inform my discussion of the purpose of circulation.

My description of Harvey's visit to Ketschin Castle is taken from Springell (1963). The quotations from Primrose at the beginning of the chapter come from French (1994).

Essay 8

My account of Descrates' ideas draws on French (1994), Russell (1946), Alberti (2010), Shapin (1996), and Fuchs (2001).

Chapter 14

Aubrey (1972) is the source for my comments on the triumph of Harvey's theory and for the Edgehill anecdote. The quotations from Harvey in this chapter are taken from Harvey (1653). My account of the Civil War draws on Worden (2009). The quotation from Charles I, regarding taxation, is taken from Keele (1965).

For my description of the changing significance of the idea of the body politic, I have drawn on I.B Cohen (1994), Hill (1964), and Shapin & Shaffer (1985). This chapter also draws on broader accounts of scientific revolution, such as those of Cohen (1985), Shapin (1996), H.F Cohen (1994), and Webster (1982; 1986).

Chapter 15

The anecdotal material in this chapter is taken from three sources: Aubrey (1972), Harvey's will (Harvey [1990]) and from the preface to Harvey (1653). Keynes (1966) is the source of the information on the library and museum at Amen Corner.

Bibliography

Ackroyd, P. *London: The Biography*. (London, 2000)

Alberti, F.B. *Matters of the Heart: History, Medicine, and Emotion*. (Oxford, 2010)

Allen, P. Medical Education in 17th-Century England. *Journal of the History of Medicine and Allied Sciences*, 1 (1946), 115–143.

Appendix to the Statutes of the College of Physicians, London, An. (London, 1696?)

Aubrey, John. *Brief Lives*. (Edited by O.L. Dick.) (Harmondsworth, 1972)

Bacon, Francis. *The Essays of Lord Bacon, including his Moral and Historical Works*. (London, 1884)

Bainvel, J.V. *Devotion to the Sacred Heart: The Doctrine and Its History*. (London, 1924)

Banyon, H.P. The Significance of the Demonstration of the Harveian Circulation by Experimental Tests. *Annals of Science*, 3 (1938), 435–446.

Barnes, B. *Scientific Knowledge and Sociological Theory*. (London, 1974)

Baron, X. (edited). *London 1066–1914: Literary Sources and Documents*. (Robertsbridge, 1997)

Basalla, G. William Harvey and the Heart as a Pump. *Bulletin of the History of Medicine*, 36 (1962), 467–470.

Bates, D.G. Harvey's Account of his "Discovery." *Journal of Medical History*, 36 (1992), 361–378.

Bayon, H.P. Allusions to a "Circulation" of the Blood in MSS Anterior to *De motu cordis* 1628. *Proceedings of the Royal Society of Medicine*, 32 (1939), 707–718.

Beier, L.M. *Sufferers and Healers: The Experience of Illness in Seventeenth Century England.* (Abingdon, 1988)

Borgherini, M. *La Vita Privata a Padova nel Secolo XVII.* (Venice, 1917)

Brockbank, W. Old Anatomical Theatres and What Took Place Therein. *Medical History*, 12 (1968), 71–84.

Brooke, C. *A History of Gonville and Caius College.* (Woodbridge, 1985)

Brooke, J.H. *Science and Religion: Some Historical Perspectives.* (Cambridge, 1991)

Burton, R. *The Anatomy of Melancholy.* (Oxford, 1989–1994)

Bylebyl, J.J. (edited). *William Harvey and his Age: The Professional and Social Context of the Discovery of the Circulation.* (Baltimore, 1979a)

Bylebyl, J.J. The Growth of Harvey's *De motu cordis. Bulletin of the History of Medicine*, 47 (1973), 427–470.

Bylebyl, J.J. The School of Padua: Humanistic Medicine in the Sixteenth Century. In *Health, Medicine and Mortality in the Sixteenth Century*, ed. Charles Webster (pp. 335–370). (Cambridge, 1979b)

Campbell, M. *The English Yeoman Under Elizabeth and the Early Stuarts.* (New Haven, 1942)

Carlino, A. *Books of the Body: Anatomical Ritual and Renaissance Learning.* (Chicago, 1999)

Chauvois, L. *William Harvey, His Life and Times: His discoveries: His Methods.* (London, 1961)

Circulation: Proceedings of the Harvey Tercentenary Congress. (Oxford, 1958)

Clark, G.N. *A History of the Royal College of Physicians of London (Vols. 1 & 2).* (Oxford, 1964)

Cohen, H.F. *The Scientific Revolution: A Historiographical Inquiry.* (Chicago, 1994)

Cohen, I.B. Harrington and Harvey: A Theory of the State Based on the New Physiology. *Journal of the History of Ideas*, 55 (1994), 187–210.

Cohen, I.B. *Revolution in Science*. (Cambridge, Mass., 1985)

Cole, F.J. *A History of Comparative Anatomy: From Aristotle to the Eighteenth Century*. (London, 1944)

Cole, F.J. Harvey's Animals. *Journal of the History of Medicine*, 12 (1957), 106–113.

Coryate, Thomas. *Coryats Crudities, 1611*. (London, 1978)

Costello, W.T. *The Scholastic Curriculum at Early Seventeenth-Century Cambridge*. (Cambridge, Mass., 1958)

Cressy, D. The Social Composition of Caius College, Cambridge 1580–1640. *Past and Present*, 47 (1970), 113–115.

Cunningham, A. William Harvey: The Discovery of the Circulation of the Blood. In *Man Masters Nature*, ed. Roy Porter (pp. 65–76) (London, 1985)

Cunningham, A. *The Anatomical Renaissance: The Resurrection of the Anatomical Projects of the Ancients*. (Aldershot, 1997)

Debus, A.G. Harvey and Fludd: The Irrational Factor in the Rational Science of the Seventeenth Century. *Journal of the History of Biology*, 3 (1970), 81–105.

Debus, A.G. *Man and Nature in the Renaissance*. (Cambridge, 1978)

Debus, A.G. Robert Fludd and the Circulation of the Blood. *Journal of the History of Medicine and Allied Sciences*, 16 (1961), 374–393.

Deep Sigh Breath'd Through the Lodgings at White-hall, A. (London, 1642)

Donne, John. *Poetry & Prose of John Donne: With Izaac Walton's "Life."* (Oxford, 1971)

Evelyn, John. *The Diary of John Evelyn*. (edited by John Bowle.) (Oxford, 1983)

Fabricius, ab Aquapendente. *De Venarum Ostiolis*. (Edited and translated by K.J. Franklin.) (Springfield, 1933)

Fabricius, ab Aquapendente. *The Embryological Treatises of Hieronymus Fabricius of Aquapendente*. (Edited and translated by H.B. Adelmann.) (Ithaca, 1942)

Feingold, M. *The Mathematicians' Apprenticeship: Science, Universities and Society in England, 1560–1640*. (Cambridge, 1984)

Ferrari, G. Public Anatomy Lessons and the Carnival: The Anatomy Theatre of Bologna. *Past and Present*, 117 (1987), 50–106.

Ferrario, E.V., & Poynter, F.N. William Harvey's Debate with Caspar Hofmann on the Circulation of the Blood. *Journal of the History of Medicine*, 15 (1960), 7–21.

Fludd, Robert. *Essential Readings*. (Edited by W.H. Hoffman.) (London, 1992)

Frank, R.G. *Harvey and the Oxford Physiologists: A Study of Scientific Ideas*. (Berkeley, 1980)

Fraser-Harris, D.F. William Harvey's Knowledge of Literature: Classical, Mediæval, Renaissance and Contemporary. *Proceedings of the Royal Society of Medicine*, 27 (1934), 1095–1099.

French, R.K. *Ancients and Moderns in the Medical Sciences: From Hippocrates to Harvey*. (Aldershot, 2000)

French, R.K. *Dissection and Vivisection in the European Renaissance*. (Aldershot, 1999)

French, R.K. *The History of the Heart: Thoracic Physiology from Ancient to Modern Times*. (Aberdeen, 1979)

French, R.K. *William Harvey's Natural Philosophy*. (Cambridge, 1994)

French, R.K., & Wear, A. (edited). *The Medical Revolution of the Seventeenth Century*. (Cambridge, 1989)

Fuchs, T. *The Mechanization of the Heart: Harvey and Descartes*. (Rochester, 2001)

Fuller, Thomas. *The History of the Worthies of England*. (London, 1662)

Guerrini, A. The Ethics of Animal Experimentation in Seventeenth-Century England. *Journal of the History of Ideas*, 50 (1989), 391–407.

Hale, D.G. *The Body Politic: A Political Metaphor in Renaissance English Literature*. (Paris, 1971)

Harvey Family. *Bloomsbury Book Auctions. Documents from the papers of Dr William Harvey (1578–1657) and Other Manuscripts and Letters*. (London, 2001)

Harvey Family. *Bloomsbury Book Auctions. Letters, Manuscripts and Historical Documents Including Further Papers of the Family of Dr*

William Harvey (1578–1657) and Other Manuscripts and Letters. (London, 2002)

Harvey, William. *Anatomical Exercitations, Concerning the Generation of Living Creatures.* (First English translation.) (London, 1653)

Harvey, William. *De Motu Locali Animalium, 1627.* (Edited and translated by G. Whitteridge.) (Cambridge, 1959)

Harvey, William. *Disputations Touching the Generation of Animals.* (Translated by G. Whitteridge.) (Oxford, 1981)

Harvey, William. *Eleven Letters of William Harvey to Lord Feilding, June 9–November 15, 1636.* (London, 1935)

Harvey, William. *Lectures on the Whole of Anatomy.* (An annotated translation by C.D. O'Malley, F.N.L. Poynter and K.F. Russell.) (Berkeley & Los Angeles, 1961)

Harvey, William. *Memorials of Harvey, including a Letter and Autographs in Facsimile.* (Collected and edited by J.H. Aveling.) (London, 1875)

Harvey, William. *Some Memoranda in Regard to William Harvey.* (Edited by S.W. Mitchell.) (New York, 1907)

Harvey, William. *Some Recently Discovered Letters of William Harvey, with Other Miscellanea.* (Edited by S.W. Mitchell.) (Philadelphia, 1912)

Harvey, William. *The Anatomical Exercises of Dr William Harvey. De Motu Cordis, 1628: De Circulatione Sanguinis, 1649.* The first English text of 1653 (edited by G. Keynes.) (London, 1928)

Harvey, William. *The Anatomical Lectures of William Harvey. Prelectiones Anatomie Universalis. De Musculis.* (Edited and translated by G. Whitteridge.) (Edinburgh and London, 1964)

Harvey, William. *The Circulation of the Blood, and Other Writings.* (Translated by K.J. Franklin, with an introduction by A. Wear.) (London, 1990)

Heilbron, J.L. *Galileo.* (Oxford, 2010)

Helfand, M.S., & Smith II, P.E. (edited). *Oscar Wilde's Oxford Notebooks: A Portrait of Mind in the Making.* (New York, 1989)

Henry, J. *Knowledge Is Power: Francis Bacon and the Method of Science.* (Cambridge, 2002)

Hesler, Baldasar. *Andreas Vesalius' First Public Anatomy at Bologna, 1540. An Eyewitness Report.* (Edited and translated by R. Eriksson.) (Stockholm, 1959)

Hill, C. William Harvey and the Idea of Monarchy. *Past and Present*, 27 (1964), 54–72.

Huffman, W.H. *Robert Fludd and the End of the Renaissance.* (London & New York, 1988)

Huntley, F. Sir Thomas Browne, M.D., William Harvey and the Metaphor of the Circle. *Bulletin of the History of Medicine*, 25 (1951), 236–247.

James, M.R. *A Descriptive Catalogue of the Manuscripts in the Library of Gonville and Caius College.* (Cambridge, 1907)

Jardine, L. *Francis Bacon: Discovery and the Art of Discourse.* (London, 1974)

Jardine, L. *Ingenious Pursuits: Building the Scientific Revolution.* (London, 1999)

Jevons, F.R. Harvey's Quantitative Method. *Bulletin of the History of Medicine*, 36 (1962), 462–467.

Journal of the Royal College of Physicians of London. (London, 1966–2000)

Jung, C.G. *The Archetypes and the Collective Unconscious.* (London, 1980)

Kearney, H.F. *Scholars and Gentlemen: Universities and Society in Pre-industrial Britain, 1500–1700.* (London, 1970)

Keele, K.D. *William Harvey: The Man, the Physician, and the Scientist.* (London, 1965)

Keynes, G. The History of Medical Practice at St Bartholomew's Hospital 1123–1700. In *The Royal Hospital of St Bartholomew 1123–1973*, ed. V.C. Medvei & J.L. Thornton (pp. 104–125). (London, 1974)

Keynes, G. *The Life of William Harvey.* (Oxford, 1966)

Keynes, G. *The Portraiture of William Harvey.* (London, 1949)

Klestinec, C. A History of Anatomy Theaters in Sixteenth-Century Padua. *Journal of the History of Medicine and Allied Sciences*, 59 (2004), 375–412.

Kuhn, T.S. *The Structure of Scientific Revolutions.* (Chicago, 1962)

Latour, B., & Woolgar. S. *Laboratory life: The Construction of Scientific Facts.* (Princeton, 1976)

LeGoff, J. Head or Heart? The Political Use of Body Metaphors in the Middle Ages. In *Fragments for a History of the Human Body (part 3),* ed. M. Feher (pp. 13–26). (London, 1989)

Letter from Queen Elizabeth to the University. In *A Collection of Letters, Statutes, and other Documents from the MS. Library of Corpus Christi College.* ed. J. Lamb (p. 278). (London, 1838)

Lind, L.R. (edited and translated). *Studies in Pre-Vesalian Anatomy.* (Philadelphia, 1975)

List of the Early Printed Books . . . in the Library of Gonville and Caius College, Cambridge, A. (Oxford, 1850)

Locke, D. *Science as Writing.* (New Haven, 1992)

Lytton Sells, A. Englishmen in Padua, from Chaucer to Shelley. *The Durham University Journal,* 9 (1947), 1–7.

Maehle A.H. The Ethical Discourse on Animal Experimentation, 1650–1900. In *Doctors and Ethics: The Earlier Historical Setting of Professional Ethics,* ed. A Wear, J. Geyer-Kordesch, & R.K. French (pp. 203–251). (Amsterdam and Atlanta, 1993)

Maehle, H., & Trohler, U. Animal Experimentation from Antiquity to the End of the Eighteenth Century: Attitudes and Arguments in Vivisection. In *Historical Perspectives,* ed. N.A. Rupke (pp. 14–47). (Croom, 1987)

Matsen, H.S. Students' "Arts" Disputations at Bologna around 1500. *Renaissance Quarterly,* 47 (1977), 533–555.

McMullen, E.T. Anatomy of a Physiological Discovery: William Harvey and the Circulation of the Blood. *Journal of the Royal Society of Medicine,* 88 (1995), 491–498.

Midgley, M. *Science and Poetry.* (London, 2001)

Moran, B.T. *Distilling Knowledge: Alchemy, Chemistry, and the Scientific Revolution.* (Cambridge, Mass., 2006)

Morgan, V., & Brooke, C. *A History of the University of Cambridge: Volume 2, 1546–1750.* (Cambridge, 2004)

Nicholl, C. *Leonardo da Vinci: The Flights of the Mind.* (London, 2005)

Nicholl, C. *The Chemical Theatre.* (London, 1980)

Nicholl, C. *The Reckoning: The Murder of Christopher Marlowe.* (London, 1992)

Nicolson, M.H. *The Breaking of the Circle. Studies in the Effect of the "New Science" upon Seventeenth-Century Poetry.* (Evanston, 1950)

O'Malley, C.D. *Andreas Vesalius of Brussels, 1514–1564.* (Berkeley, 1964)

Ongaro, G., Maurizio R.B., & Gaetano, T. (edited). *Harvey e Padova: Atti del Convegno Celebrativo del Quarto Centenario della Laurea di William Harvey, 2002.* (Treviso, 2006)

Pagel, W. *New Light on William Harvey.* (Basel, 1976)

Pagel, W. The Philosophy of Circles-Cesalpino-Harvey. A Penultimate Assessment. *Journal of the History of Medicine,* 12 (1957), 140–157.

Pagel, W. William Harvey and the Purpose of Circulation. *Isis,* 42 (1951), 22–38.

Pagel, W. *William Harvey's Biological Ideas.* (Basel, 1967)

Park, K. The Criminal and Saintly Body: Autopsy and Dissection in Renaissance Italy. *Renaissance Quarterly,* 47 (1994), 1–33.

Park, K., Daston, L.J., Lindberg, D.C., & Numbers, R.L. (edited). *The Cambridge History of Science: Early Modern Science* (Volume 3). (Cambridge, 2003)

Payne, F.J. *Notes to Accompany a Facsimile Reproduction of the Diploma of Doctor of Medicine Granted by the University of Padua to William Harvey 1602.* (London, 1908)

Payne, L.E.S. *With Words and Knives: Learning Medical Dispassion in Early Modern England.* (Aldershot, 2007)

Payne, L.M. Sir Charles Scarburgh's Harveian Oration, 1662. *Journal of the History of Medicine and Allied Sciences,* 12 (1957), 158–164.

Pazzini, A. William Harvey, Disciple of Girolamo Fabrizi d'Acquapendente and the Paduan School. *Journal of the History of Medicine,* 12 (1957), 197–201.

Picard, L. *Elizabeth's London: Everyday Life in Elizabethan London.* (London, 2003)

Power, D'Arcy. *William Harvey*. (London, 1897)

Poynter, F.N. John Donne and William Harvey. *Journal of the History of Medicine and Allied Sciences*, 15 (1960), 233–246.

Pritchard, R.E. *Shakespeare's England: Life in Elizabethan and Jacobean Times*. (Stroud, 1999)

Prockter, A. *The A to Z of Elizabethan London*. (London, 1979)

Randall, J.H. The Development of Scientific Method in the School of Padua. *Journal of the History of Ideas*, 1 (1940), 177–206.

Randall, J.H. *The School of Padua: And the Emergence of Modern Science*. (Padua, 1961)

Richards, S. *Philosophy and Sociology of Science: An Introduction*. (Oxford, 1983)

Rupp, J.C.C. Matters of Life and Death, the Social and Cultural Conditions of the Rise of Anatomical Theatres. *History of Science*, 28 (1990), 263–287.

Russell, B. *History of Western Philosophy: And Its Connection with Political and Social Circumstances from the Earliest Times to the Present Day*. (London, 1946)

Sawday, J. *The Body Emblazoned: Dissection and the Human Body in Renaissance Culture*. (London, 1995)

Schmitt, C.B. *Aristotle and the Renaissance*. (Cambridge, Mass., 1983)

Shapin, S. *A Social History of Truth: Civility and Science in Seventeenth-Century England*. (Chicago, 1994)

Shapin, S. The House of Experiment in Seventeenth-Century England. *Isis*, 79 (1988), 373–404.

Shapin, S. *The Scientific Revolution*. (Chicago, 1996)

Shapin, S., & Schaffer, S. *Leviathan and the Air-Pump: Hobbes, Boyle, and the Experimental Life*. (Princeton, 1985)

Shugg, W. Humanitarian Attitudes in the Early Animal Experiments of the Royal Society. *Annals of Science*, 24 (1968), 227–238.

Singer, C. *A Short History of Anatomy and Physiology from the Greeks to Harvey*. (New York, 1957)

Sloan, A.W. *English Medicine in the Seventeenth Century*. (Durham, 1996)

Springell, F.C. (edited). *Connoisseur & Diplomat: The Earl of Arundel's Embassy to Germany in 1636 as Recounted in William Crowne's Diary, the Earl's Letters, and Other Contemporary Sources.* (London, 1963)

Statutes of Queen Elizabeth for the University of Cambridge. Translated from the original Latin statutes. (London, 1838)

Stow, John. *The Survey of London.* (London, 1956)

Thomas, K. *Religion and the Decline of Magic: Studies in Popular Beliefs in Sixteenth and Seventeenth Century England.* (London, 1971)

Thomas, K. *The Ends of Life: Roads to Fulfilment in Early Modern England.* (Oxford, 2009)

Thompson, C.J.S. *The Quacks of Old London.* (New York, 1928)

Tillyard, E.M.W. *The Elizabethan World Picture.* (London, 1943)

Traister, B.H. *The Notorious Astrological Physician of London: Works and Days of Simon Forman.* (Chicago, 2001)

Underwood, E.A. The Early Teaching of Anatomy at Padua (with a Model of the Paduan Anatomy Theatre). *Annals of Science,* 19 (1963), 1–26.

Valenze, D.M. *The Social Life of Money in the English Past.* (Cambridge, 2006)

Venn, J. *Caius College.* (London, 1901)

Vesalius, Andreas. *The Epitome of Andreas Vesalius.* (Translated by L.R. Lind, anatomical notes by C.W. Asling.) (New York, 1949)

Wear, A. *Knowledge and Practice in English Medicine, 1550–1680.* (Cambridge, 2000)

Wear, A. William Harvey and the "Way of the Anatomists." *History of Science,* 21 (1983), 223–249.

Wear, A., French, R.K., & Lonie, I.M. (edited). *The Medical Renaissance of the Sixteenth Century.* (Cambridge, 1985)

Webster, C. *From Paracelsus to Newton: Magic and the Making of Modern Science.* (Cambridge, 1982)

Webster, C. *The Great Instauration: Science, Medicine and Reform, 1626–1660.* (New York, 1986)

Whitteridge, G. *William Harvey and the Circulation of the Blood.* (London, 1971)

Wilson, L. William Harvey's Prelectiones: The Performance of the Body in the Renaissance Theater of Anatomy. *Representations*, 17 (1987), 62–95.

Woolfson, J. *Padua and the Tudors: English Students in Italy, 1485–1603.* (Toronto, 1998)

Worden, B. *The English Civil Wars, 1640–1660.* (London, 2009)

Young J.R. Poetical Allusions to the Circulation of Blood up to the End of the Seventeenth Century. *Vesalius: Acta internationales historiae medicinae*, 9 (2003), 3–8.

Further Reading

ANYONE WISHING TO read a conventional chronological account of Harvey's 'life and times' can turn to Keynes' *Life*. Easily surpassing his predecessors, Power and Chauvois, Keynes is meticulous and exhaustive as a biographer. I have relied on his vast mine of information throughout the compilation of this book.

To twenty-first-century eyes, however, the account of Harvey's quest offered by Keynes (and also by his predecessors) appears anachronistic, animated as it is by the positivistic and 'Whiggish' beliefs of the nineteenth and twentieth centuries—the idea that authentic knowledge can only be arrived at through experiment and the senses; and the conviction that the store of 'scientific' knowledge accumulates with time, and so ensures human progress. Keynes, like his precursors, presents Harvey as an empirical scientist, and as a thoroughly rational man, whose research proceeded logically, on a sort of inevitable progress towards truth.

Over the last fifty years, this traditional interpretation of Harvey's quest has been revised, or rejected outright, by a number of Harvey scholars. Andrew Cunningham, Roger French, Andrew Wear and Walter Pagel (to name the foremost experts) have produced far more nuanced, historically sensitive and intellectually interesting analyses of Harvey's endeavour. I have drawn widely on their impressive body of work throughout; without it, indeed, this book could not have been written. I recommend to the curious and intrepid general reader the works of these academics, who succeed in discussing complex and sometimes esoteric subjects in a style that is clear and accessible. As the price of their scholarly books is generally prohibitive, however, I encourage readers to try to track them down at public libraries—presuming that their local libraries remain open. Anyone interested in reading a general account of 'science' in the seventeenth century should consult Steven Shapin's excellent introduction, or Lisa Jardine's *Ingenious Pursuits*, while those curious about scientific revolutions can read Thomas Kuhn's classic work on the subject.

Finally, I would urge anyone interested in Harvey to read *De motu cordis* itself, in Kenneth Franklin's lucid modern translation, which has been published in paperback by Everyman with an introduction by Andrew Wear. Harvey's masterpiece can be enjoyed not only as an account of his researches, and of the formulation of his great theory, but also as a fine and fascinating work of seventeenth-century literature and philosophy. His clear, vivid prose returns us to a time in which 'science' was a sister study to 'humanities' disciplines, and benefited profoundly from that close relationship.

List of Illustrations

Index